HOW TO COPE
SUCCESSFULLY WITH
DIVERTICULITIS

DR JOAN MCCLELLAND

Wellhouse Publishing Ltd

First published in Great Britain in 2001 by
Wellhouse Publishing Ltd
31 Middle Bourne Lane
Lower Bourne
Farnham
Surrey GU10 3NH

Reprinted in 2003 (Twice)

DISCLAIMER

The aim of this book is to provide general information only and should
not be treated as a substitute for the medical advice of your doctor or
any other health care professional. The publisher and author is not
responsible or liable for any diagnosis made by a reader based on the
contents of this book. Always consult your doctor if you are in any way
concerned about your health.

A catalogue record for this book is available from the British Library

ISBN 1 903784 00 X

Printed and bound in Great Britain by
Biddles Ltd., Surrey. www.biddles.co.uk

Contents

Introduction

Two women were sitting in front of me on the bus.

'Diverticular disease? I've never heard of it.'

'Well, that's what the doctor says my mother's got. I don't know whether to take it seriously, or whether it's psychosomatic.'

'How does it affect her?'

'That's the point. It doesn't. She seems perfectly OK apart from the odd tummy-ache. She's a bit overweight - but who isn't at 60-plus - and, of course, she's always suffered from constipation. I tell her she ought to eat more greens.'

'How did they find out about it, if she wasn't having any symptoms?'

'It was quite by chance. She'd had a bit of trouble with piles and they did an X-ray just to check, and that's when they saw the signs of the diverticular disease. Apparently the piles were a clue, and lots of people have it without knowing.'

'I can't see it matters, in that case. Still, it gives your mother something to talk about.'

'*She* says she knows of someone who nearly died of it, but, as I said...'

The bus stopped and the women got off, still talking, and I did not hear any more. But it had set me thinking. I was longing to tell them just why diverticular disease *does* matter, and why people ought to know about it.

Chapter One

What It Is and Why It Matters

The Gastroenterology Clinic (GUTS among friends) was crowded, as usual. I knew that as many as half the people my colleagues and I would see would have problems associated with diverticular disease. I wished that the ladies on the bus could have been there, so that I could have had a chance of giving them the facts. This is what I would have told them -

- Diverticular disease involves definite changes in the structure of the bowel - and there is nothing psychosomatic about that.
- It is so widespread that each of us stands a more than 50 per cent chance of getting it by the time we reach 60, but we may not always realize that we have got it.
- Although it may cause nothing worse than a little abdominal discomfort which you may brush aside, it has the potential to spring an emergency on you, at any time.

Diverticular disease is very common, can be dangerous, and is increasing rapidly, but it gets almost no media attention. There are one hundred people suffering from diverticular disease for *every* one with Crohn's disease. Yet the latter is always in the news and diverticular disease is neglected.

The Digestive Disorders Foundation, a charity that promotes research into digestive problems, recently did something to redress the balance. They organized a major conference on diverticular disease. Two of us from the clinic attended it. Sufferers and others involved, as well as doctors, made up the audience - and it was the sufferers who asked the most searching and interesting questions.

What Is Diverticular Disease?

Diverticula (singular: *diverticulum*) are little pockets of gut lining that bulge out through the wall of the digestive tube. They can crop up anywhere along its length, but 90 per cent occur in the large intestine, or colon. Any problems associated with these diverticula come under the umbrella of *diverticular disease*, most properly called *diverticular disease of the colon*.

Broadly, diverticular disease comprises two conditions:

Diverticulosis always comes first. It just means the presence of diverticula.

A minimum of three diverticula are needed to make the diagnosis, but usually there are many more.

Diverticulitis involves inflammation and often infection of some of the diverticula.

As with arthrosis and arthritis, the version ending in *-osis* refers to simple 'wear and tear' effects, while the *-itis* ending indicates inflammation, as in appendic*itis* or tonsill*itis*.

While diverticul*osis* may cause some pain or discomfort, it is often completely 'silent'; you may not even know you have got it. In this situation the diagnosis is tricky and, as with the mother of the woman on the bus, it may only show up by chance. Diverticul*itis*, by contrast, is always painful and may also produce other symptoms.

Diverticulosis: often no symptoms
Diverticulitis: always painful, sometimes other symptoms
20-25 per cent of those with diverticulosis progress to diverticulitis.

Dangers arise when extra problems set in. For instance, in 1989, 1,480 people in England and Wales died because of complications related to diverticular disease. The death rate has increased steadily, year on year, since the beginning of the 20th century - apart from a significant standstill from 1939-45, when a restricted national diet was in force.

Who Is at Risk?

We may be able to reduce our personal risk if we understand the causes of the illness, and the preventative measures that can help.

Sex
The sexes come out roughly equal overall, but aged under 50 you are slightly more susceptible if you are a man, and aged 50 and over, women are more at risk. This trend is enhanced now we are all living longer, with women living even longer than men.

Age
Since diverticular disease is due to an age-related weakening of the muscles of the colon, the likelihood of having diverticular disease increases steadily as you get older. In fact, we are all likely to develop diverticula unless we die young, but we may never develop the symptoms of the disease.

Age Table

Under 30	⇨	Rare
Under 40	⇨	Uncommon
45 and over	⇨	30% are affected
70 and over	⇨	50% are affected
80 and over	⇨	60% are affected
85 and over	⇨	80% are affected

Note: these percentages apply only in affluent countries like the US and UK.

Where You Live

The whole of the adult population living in the modern Western culture is 50-100 times more likely to develop diverticular disease than those in rural Africa or Asia. People living in North America, the UK and Western Europe, Australia and New Zealand and those who share their technologically assisted lifestyle are the most at risk.

National Statistics
Numbers affected

USA	25% of the total population
UK	10% or more of the total population (more than 50% of those over 70)
Africa and Asia	0.2% of the population (apart from the urban wealthy)
Israel	Jewish population - as in the USA Arab population - many fewer
South Africa	Whites - as in Western cultures Blacks and people of colour - as in the rest of Africa
Japan	Westernized lifestyle - as in Western cultures Traditional lifestyle - as in rural Asia
Hawaii	First-generation Japanese - as in the traditional figures Subsequent generations - approaching the USA statistics
Singapore	- stands out as a place where diverticular disease is escalating in parallel with the increasingly affluent standard of living

Note
Doctors Burkitt and Painter, who spent 20 years in Uganda, and became famous for their work on bowel disorders, did not find a single case of diverticular disease, and on enquiring from colleagues all over Africa, unearthed only two cases over the same period. They made their report in 1969.

*When*You Live
Diverticular disease is, without doubt, a disorder of the 20th and 21st centuries, and the numbers continue to increase.

Admissions to hospital for diverticular disease and its complications: *Scotland*: between 1960 and 1970 the number of people hospitalized for diverticular disease doubled

4% of all hospital admissions in the UK among the over-65s were for diverticular disease - in the 1990s

17% of Medicare cases in the US were due to diverticular disease and its complications - also in the 1990s

The upward trend continues.

If you live in the Western countries of America, Western Europe and Australia, the way to achieve a low-risk situation would be by travelling back in time - at least 100 years. There was very little diverticular disease in these countries in 1920 compared with 1990, and the trend continues to get worse. The alternative is to choose the simple life, and so reduce your chance of developing diverticular disease - or more probably the risk to your children.

Why Is the Situation Getting Worse?

You might think that with all the wealth and welfare, technological, pharmaceutical and medical know-how and the blueprint of human life, the human genome itself, unfolded before us, we in this modern Western culture would be the least likely to succumb to an illness such as diverticular disease, or to be unable to control it. You would be quite wrong.

The facts are inescapable. There is something in our feather-bedded lifestyle that sets us up for diverticular disease, among a host of other nasties, such as coronary disease, hiatus hernia, gallstones, varicose veins, obesity, colon cancer and diabetes. Saint's Triad is the name given to a common grouping of three illnesses: diverticular disease, hiatus hernia, and gallstones, which affect 6 per cent of the over-65s.

What Are We Doing Wrong?

The biggest difference between the way we live now and the way we lived in times past is what we eat and the physical effort involved in getting it. The more remote parts of the developing world are in a time warp in these respects.

The agricultural revolution, when growing crops largely took over from herding animals, was the first step towards the supermarket culture. The effects of the Industrial Revolution were even more dramatic. Machines began increasingly to replace muscle power, throughout the Victorian era. Less exercise meant softer muscles, all over, including those of the gut. Fresh foods were gradually replaced by processed and refined products, preserved by canning or chemicals. A most far-reaching change was the introduction of the roller-milling of flour in 1880.

This ushered in the age of cheap and easy wheat and cereal foods, made palatable with pure, sweet, refined white sugar: buns, bagels, cakes and pasta and soft, sliced bread, and breakfast cereals. Digesting these is easy - and so is putting on excess weight - and since these foods provide the minimum of indigestible waste, the colon has, literally, very little to get a grip on. The large well-muscled colon of the African country-dweller has a smaller, weaker counterpart in first-world man and woman.

It is significant that the death rate from disease of the colon increased sharply from around 1910, when enough time had elapsed for a new generation to have been brought up on soft, sweet, refined foods. Similarly, diverticular disease stopped increasing during the period of the Second World War when bread was rationed, and the National Loaf was 85 per cent wholemeal.

Constipation was no problem to our forbears, but today it is common and in particular a bane to the elderly, whose colonic muscles are naturally less strong. It is an important element in the development of diverticular disease.

How Did Diverticular Disease Start?

Like other disorders and malfunctions, diverticular disease is the end-result of a chain of bodily events, including injuries and infections, dietary and other habits, and changes associated with living conditions and age. Since a major factor in the development of diverticular disease is wear and tear in the ageing colon, there must always have been some cases of the disorder. These would probably have been among the rich and successful who would depend less on large quantities of vegetables, because they would be able to afford the more concentrated nourishment of meat, fish and cheese. Interestingly, instances of disorder of the bowel are recorded as early as 1700 BC. For those who are interested, I include a brief history of the condition on page 123.

Detecting Diverticular Disease

Seeing the inside of the whole of the colon, including diverticula and any other abnormality, is now standard practice. Nevertheless, exactly how the colon works still holds some puzzles.

New methods of visualizing the colon without physical intrusion have now been developed. Today we have a wealth of imaging techniques, from barium enema to magnetic resonance, together with endoscopy and fibreoptics, to help ensure that the colon can hide no secrets. They are particularly valuable in cases of infection, when introducing an endoscope might make matters worse. Two forms of X-ray provide 3-D images: the CAT scan (Computerized Axial Tomography) and MRI (Magnetic Resonance Imaging), and the entirely harmless ultrasound, developed in the 1950s.

Chapter Two

Anatomy and Physiology

For many, it helps to understand how the bowel and the digestive system work, and so this chapter offers a brief explanation.

The digestive system consists of one very long tube, from the mouth to the anus - 30 feet or 9 metres long - with food entering at one end, waste matter exiting at the other. The part that is involved in diverticular disease is the *colon*, or large intestine or large bowel. It is the last important stretch of gut before the waste disposal unit at the end. Seen from the front, it is arranged like this.

Diagram 1

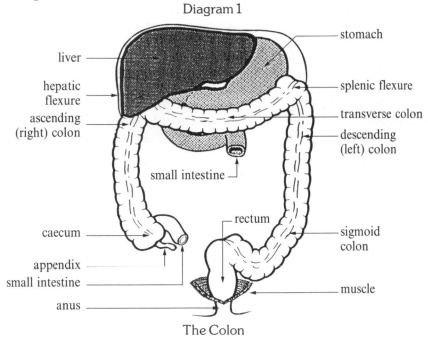

The Colon

In the upper left corner of the diagram (top right in your body) is the liver. It is tucked in under the ribs, just below the diaphragm, the sheet of muscle separating the chest from the abdomen. The liver overlaps the stomach, which is on your left side, and also one corner of the colon. The colon is partly covered by the coils of the small intestine, but these have been omitted from the diagram, to show the colon more clearly.

	Length	Width
Small intestine	6.7 m (22 ft)	50 mm (2 in) at the beginning
		25 mm (1 in) at the end
Large intestine	1.5 m (4 ft 11 in)	10 cm (4 in)

The small intestine is much narrower than the large intestine, and joins onto it low down on your right. A valve called the *ileocaecal valve* (not shown) prevents the contents of the colon flowing back into the small intestine. The colon starts with a bulge called the *caecum* (Latin for 'blind alley'). Sticking out of that is the appendix, a little cul-de-sac of gut representing the vestiges of an organ for digesting grass. Horses have well-developed appendices, but they are of no known use to modern man and are occasionally a danger. If an infection sets up in the appendix, since it has no free drainage, acute inflammation (acute appendicitis) may result, with a risk of perforation or bursting. Diverticula are like mini-appendices, and they too can become severely inflamed and even perforate.

Running up from the caecum is the *ascending colon*, ending in the *hepatic flexure* behind the liver (*hepatic* means to do with the liver). The colon now loops across the body from right to left. This is the *transverse colon*, ending in the *splenic flexure*, next to the spleen. Next comes the *descending colon*, running down the left side of your abdomen. The last part is called the *sigmoid colon*, so called because it twists round like an 'S', from the Greek *sigma*.

Diagram 2

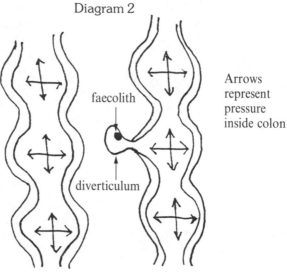

faecolith

diverticulum

Arrows represent pressure inside colon

Longitudinal Section of the Colon

The sigmoid colon is especially important because more than 90 per cent of diverticula crop up in this small area and any pain from diverticular disease is almost always low down on the left, like appendicitis pain, but on the wrong side. Odd diverticula can arise anywhere along the digestive tube, as a developmental quirk, but diverticular disease is a disorder of the colon. It is rare in the caecum, ascending and transverse colons, and uncommon in the descending colon until it reaches the sigmoid stretch.

The pressure inside the gut becomes progressively higher, the nearer it is to the anus, and the colon is especially constructed to maximize this. This pressure is of critical importance in diverticular disease.

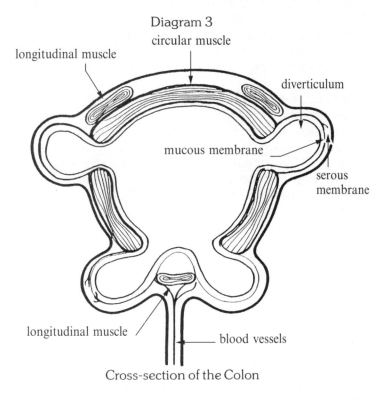

Diagram 3

Cross-section of the Colon

Instead of being a simple tube like a hosepipe, the colon consists of a series of interconnecting compartments, each separated from the next by a constricting ring of muscle, like an elastic belt. Each segment builds up its own internal pressure and the result can be as high as the equivalent of 90 mm of mercury. This is useful for compressing the contents of the colon into a convenient consistency, but has the major disadvantage of tending to produce diverticula. They are more likely to form as the supporting tissues begin to lose their *elastin* and *collagen* with increasing age - an effect you can see in your surface skin. Bags, sags and wrinkles are the tell-tale signs.

The tensile strength of the colon, that is, its ability to regain its shape after being stretched, like a fabric with Lycra, is at its highest before you are ten years old!

The muscles of the colon comprise two types: circular and longitudinal. The circular muscles in particular are responsible for the waves of constriction known as *peristalsis* which propel the food waste on towards the anus. The longitudinal muscles consist of three strong strips which limit how far the colon stretches longways. All these muscles get thicker with the advancing years. This is especially noticeable in diverticular disease, when the thickened muscle may partially block the passageway down the middle of the colon. It also tends to be stiffer, with no 'give'. This throws a strain on the weakest places in the colon wall, for instance where the blood vessels enter. Transit of the motions down the colon is also slowed up.

The inside of the bowel is lined with mucous membrane, similar to that inside your mouth, except that it is insensitive to touch, or even being cut, in common with the lining of the whole gut as far as the anus. This membrane (*mucosa*) produces a jelly-like lubricant, mucus, to ease the way of the motions. More mucus is poured out in response to irritation. *The mucosa is easily stretched, and bulges out if it is not supported by muscle - this is the situation with a diverticulum.*

The insensitivity of its lining does not mean that you *cannot* get pain from your bowel, but it is set off by stretching, distension, muscle spasm or an infection. The intestines only give you a vague idea of which part the pain is coming from, but that does not prevent it from doubling you up.

The outside of the colon is wrapped in a fold of the *peritoneum*, the membrane that lines the whole abdomen. Inflammation of the peritoneum, *peritonitis*, is a serious condition which can arise as a complication of diverticular disease.

How the Colon Works

Every part of the digestive system has its part to play, in synchrony with the rest. The sight, smell or even the thought of food is enough to activate the digestion. Your mouth waters - that is, it produces a flow of saliva which lubricates the food and, later, rinses your mouth. It also contains an enzyme for digesting starchy foods, like bread and potatoes.

Advance warning of food on the way down is flashed to all parts of the digestive tract. In particular the *gastro-colic reflex* sends a message to the colon when a meal arrives in the stomach - a useful reminder to get rid of any waste matter ready for disposal, so as to free up space in the digestive tract. The common practice of going to the toilet shortly after breakfast illustrates this.

The usual transit time between food entering the system and waste leaving it is 36-48 hours. Food is smashed up roughly in the mouth and churned up in the stomach, so that it is thoroughly mixed with the digestive juices and stomach acid. The capacity of the stomach is 1.25 litres (2-and-a-quarter pints), and it is here that the proteins - meat, fish and cheese - are mainly digested, that is, converted into a form that the body can absorb.

In the first reaches of the small intestine, including the duodenum, the pancreas and liver release their juices, to deal with fats and oils in the diet. The digestion of protein and starch continues. The contents of the gut are by now like runny porridge, and in the lower part of the small intestine, the *ileum*, the nourishing ingredients of the food are absorbed.

The outflow from the ileum is practically liquid and amounts to about a litre (2 pints) by the time it goes through the ileocaecal valve, into the caecum and then to the ascending colon.

The Main Tasks of the Colon

1. *Removal of water* from the colon contents, together with some chemicals, by the selective action of the mucosa. Cellulose or fibre, the indigestible part of plants, passes unchanged through the digestive processing and it also retains water, so a high-fibre diet means a bulkier motion. This is an insurance against constipation.

2. *Conveying the waste matter towards the anus.* A network of nerves and various hormones control the squeezing movements of the colon. Eating a meal boosts the motility of the colon considerably, and you may be aware of this. When you go to sleep the colon takes a rest, too, and its muscle activity falls off. It revs up again as soon as you wake up.
    - *Mental stress* increases the movements of the colon.
    - *Drugs* may either stimulate or inhibit the gut. For example, laxatives like senna loosen the bowels to the point of diarrhoea, while tranquillizers like Largactil cause constipation.

3. *Storage of the motions* until it is convenient to pass them. The rectum is the last section of the large intestine. It is normally empty, and when material enters it you feel the urge to go to the toilet. The average amount passed daily is 150 ml (5 fl.oz). The anus, or exit, is closed by a double ring of muscle, the internal and external sphincters, a fail-safe arrangement to prevent accidents.

How Diverticula Arise

The basic cause of diverticula is raised pressure inside the bowel finding a weak spot in the wall. The sigmoid colon is by far the most often affected because here the colon is at its narrowest and the pressure highest. Waves, or pulses, of extra high pressure are generated in the separate compartments of the bowel (see Diagram 2, p. 12). The thick muscle layer fails to relax and the brunt is borne by the vulnerable areas, especially where the blood vessels come in and the soft, stretchy mucous lining is unsupported except by the thin outer covering of the colon. It bulges out between the muscles, forming a pocket.

From the inside of the colon only a slit-like entrance is seen, but on the outside there is a little lump. Diverticula range in size from 0.5-1.0 cm (one-sixth to one-third of an inch) in diameter, and tend to be arranged in rows between the longitudinal muscle bands (the taeniae).

An uncommon complication of diverticular disease is the presence of giant sigmoid diverticula. They may be several centimetres (up to 3 inches) in diameter. They are formed by gas becoming trapped, and show up on X-ray as large, round, see-through shadows. They look very much like balloons, which is exactly what they are. Like other diverticula, they may produce no symptoms. On the other hand, if they become inflamed, they may advertise their presence by abdominal pain, a raised temperature and a swelling you can feel.

ChapterThree

Constipation

Constipation is often a significant indicator of the presence of diverticular disease, along with bleeding from the back passage and other various pains. Frequently it shows up after an X-ray or ultrasound for something quite different. It is likely that constipation is the key problem in diverticular disease, both before it develops and after.

Margaret had been troubled with constipation as long as she could remember, and she was now 58. She had good and bad days, but it had gradually been getting worse, especially over the last 18 months. Now she had a struggle most days in spite of eating bran cereal for breakfast and an apple a day. Her GP had sent her for some lab tests 'to be on the safe side' in view of her age.

The significance of her age was that the over-40s, and in particular the over-50s, are in the cancer age range. The doctor wanted to check that there was no question of, for instance, colon cancer. This is a common disorder, but with the proper treatment it does not need to shorten life. In Margaret's case the likelihood of her constipation being due to anything serious was minuscule, if it had really been going on since her teens.

The medical registrar went through all the causes of constipation. The following questions are commonly asked:

Preliminary Questions

1. First, is it truly constipation? (Did Margaret pass a motion fewer than four times a week, and/or was it hard and difficult to pass, sometimes in rocky lumps, at least a quarter of the time?)
2. Is this a sudden, acute problem or a chronic condition? (In Margaret's case it was definitely chronic.)
3. Is passing a motion painful? (For Margaret it was sometimes difficult and uncomfortable but not really painful, so it was not due to inflamed piles or a fissure - crack in the anus.)
4. Is there plenty of fibre in the diet - fruit, vegetables and bran products? Is the person drinking enough, say one-and-a-half to two litres a day?
5. Is the person taking enough exercise? For example, a brisk 40-minute walk three or four times a week as a minimum? A scramble to work on the tube, then a sedentary job with a word processor can leave one too tired to feel like a session at the gym after work, and your muscles,

inside and out, become slack and inefficient.

6. Immobilized? It is a killer - to muscle power if you have an illness like flu, or break a leg so that you are unable to move around in the ordinary way for a week or more. It is even worse if you have a long-term problem such as arthritis to slow you up, or a partial paralysis or weakness (hemiplegia) after a stroke.

7. Are you in such a rush in the mornings (getting the kids to school, getting ready for work, etc.) that you put off going to the toilet even though your bowel tells you it is ready? If you ignore it too often your bowel will give up sending you the message, and will get bunged up.

8. Have you another illness confusing the issue? For instance, could your constipation be a symptom of underactive thyroid (hypothyroidism), too much calcium in the blood (hypercalcaemia), depression or any of a handful of disorders of the colon?

9. Finally, review any medicines you take regularly or often. Some of those that cause constipation are:

Painkillers, the stronger the worse
Tranquillizers and theValium-type drugs for anxiety
Sleeping tablets
Anti-inflammatories for joint and other pains
Antacids, especially those containing aluminium or calcium
Antidepressants
Water tablets (diuretics)
Antispasmodics and anticholinergics
Blood pressure medicines
Drugs for Parkinson's disease
Contraceptive pill
Iron pills

There was no doubt about the primary diagnosis for Margaret. It was, as she said, constipation. The next step was to find the cause. Since it had begun so many years before, the chances were that it was the result of a poor diet over a long period of time, and too little exercise. Nevertheless, it did no harm to consider the possibilities.

Causes of Constipation

1. *Disorders of the anus and rectum* - such as piles, tumour or ulcer of the rectum, or an extra narrow anus (anal stenosis), sometimes due to an infection.

2. *Problems in the pelvis* - mainly female: pregnancy and the recovery period after the birth, ovarian cyst, tumour of the ovary or womb, or endometriosis, a disorder starting in the lining of the womb.
3. *Neuromuscular disorders* - that is, of the nerves or muscles of the gut. Examples include Hirschsprung's disease, a congenitally large, baggy colon; the effects of a stroke or multiple sclerosis on the nerves to the gut; systemic sclerosis and some other rarities.
4. *Endocrine or glandular diseases* - diabetes, underactive thyroid or a pituitary disorder. Margaret's thyroxine level was borderline low, which may have been a factor in her constipation.
5. *Metabolic abnormalities* - lead poisoning, shortage of potassium, porphyria, or kidney failure.
6. *Psychological problems* - the only relevant one is depression, not just unhappiness but a general damping down of vitality including sluggishness of the bowels. Margaret was mildly depressed, not badly enough to be a main cause of her constipation, but tending to make it worse.
7. *Environmental situation* - general weakness, such as follows an illness; dehydration from any cause - even hot weather; immobilization; postoperative state - temporary; the awkwardness and embarrassment of bedpans.
8. *Drugs and medicines* - listed above; also prolonged or excessive use of laxatives, until the bowel no longer responds to the stimulus of the purgative. Margaret was already finding that she needed increasing doses of the stimulant laxatives to achieve a result.
9. *Colon disorders* - these are obviously the likeliest to cause constipation, headed by the irritable colon syndrome and diverticular disease. Others to exclude are colon cancer, ulcerative colitis, Crohn's disease and abdominal tuberculosis.

Margaret's diverticular disease was diagnosed for certain by a *double contrast barium enema* (see Chapter Eight). It can sometimes be difficult to distinguish between diverticular disease and a tumour from the barium X-ray. In either case constipation may be the only symptom. A fail-safe method of ensuring the diagnosis is *colonoscopy*, looking at the whole of the inside of the colon with a fibreoptic endoscope (see Chapter Eight). This is sometimes difficult if the colon happens to be narrow and twisty in places and can be dangerous in acute diverticulitis or when there is an abscess.

In Margaret's case the barium enema provided sufficient information for a firm secondary diagnosis of diverticular disease, as well as the primary diagnosis of chronic constipation.

The Impact on the Body of Chronic Constipation

Constipation is the invariable forerunner of diverticular disease. This means that all the causes of long-term constipation are indirectly causes of diverticular disease. *Anismus* is a type of constipation, commonest in young women, in which the anal sphincter, the ring of muscle, which closes off the rectum, does not relax properly at the appropriate time. This means the abdominal and gut muscles have to push hard against the sphincter muscle to pass a motion.

Constipation, including anismus, which involves straining to pass a motion, increases the pressure inside the lower, sigmoid part of the colon in particular. The lining membrane may pop out through any weak places in the colon wall forming diverticula.

Avoiding Constipation - or Dealing with It

The basic requirements are a high-fibre diet and plenty of fluid (not alcoholic), backed up by a healthy lifestyle (see over).

A high-fibre diet on its own may not be enough to deal with established constipation at first, especially in the case of the very elderly, or weak. In these situations laxatives may be necessary, albeit on a temporary basis if possible.

Laxatives
1. *Bulk laxatives*: act by filling the rectum and setting off the reflex for passing a motion. Examples are *Fybogel* and *Regulan*, containing ispaghula husk, *Normacol*, containing sterculia, and *Celevac*, containing methylcellulose.
2. *Stimulant laxatives*: increase the movements of the bowel and may cause colic. Used long term, they lose their efficacy. Senna preparations are the mildest. Others are *Dulcolax*, containing bisacodyl, and castor oil.
3. *Softeners*: make the motion easier to pass. Examples are *Norgalax*, *Micralax*. Liquid paraffin has disadvantages and dangers.
4. *Osmotic laxatives*: work by drawing fluid into the bowel. You must take plenty of water with them. Lactulose preparations are preferable to sodium salts.
5. *Medication via the back passage*: includes suppositories and enemas.

Lifestyle
Regular high-fibre meals and regular exercise are the basis for regular action of the bowels. Problems can arise with:

- Irregular meals
- Shift work
- Inadequate or unpleasant toilet facilities
- Poor teeth so that raw fruit and vegetables, and meat, are difficult to eat

The Outcome for Margaret
Thyroxine tablets corrected Margaret's borderline hypothyroidism long term. She was not given an antidepressant for her low mood, as this type of medication would have worsened her constipation, increasing the likelihood of her current diverticulosis producing more complex symptoms. In any case, the thyroxine and improvement in her constipation lifted her spirits. Overhaul of her lifestyle was the best way to prevent the worsening of her diverticular disorder and to avoid the development of acute episodes of inflammation - diverticulitis.

Her family doctor monitors her progress now, with a gastroenterology department available whenever she may need it.

Chapter Four

Bleeding

Blood - red for danger - is always frightening when it's somewhere it shouldn't be, but one in three of the sufferers of diverticular disease bleed at some time. It can be the first sign of the disease.

Jenny was 52 years old, 1.6 metres (5 ft 4 inches) tall and nudging 69 kg (11 stone), with three kids at university. She had noticed blood on her toilet paper more than once. The first time she had ignored it, but the second and third episodes put her in a panic, especially as it was getting worse and sometimes staining her underwear. The doctor was reassuring from the start, but congratulated her on her good sense in coming for advice.

A PR (per rectum) examination with a gloved finger in the anus showed that she had a large pile which was the source of the blood, bright red because it was fresh. Haemorrhoids are so common that just because someone has them it does not mean that they cannot have any other condition. Because of her age - over 50, and so in the cancer risk group - Jenny went through all the investigations for diagnosing the cause of gastrointestinal bleeding.

Jack was 62, red-faced and jolly, with a liking for single malt whisky. One morning he had woken up with a sudden urge to go to the toilet. He was shocked to see that he had passed a large, dark-red motion, and he felt quite shaky. This is typical of diverticular disease. The bleeding usually stops spontaneously, as it did in Jack's case, but since there is a 30 per cent risk of its recurring, it is vital to find out exactly where it came from.

Possible Causes of Lower Gastrointestinal Haemorrhage (Bleeding from the Colon or Rectum)

Affecting Any Age
Haemorrhoids
Haemorrhoids are folds of redundant or spare mucosa (or mucous membrane) found at or near the anus. They are also known as piles. Until recently it was thought that haemorrhoids were varicose veins, although this did not make medical sense. It is now realized that they consist of folds of loose membrane lining the part just inside the anus. This extra membrane is needed to accommodate, temporarily, a big hard lump of waste material (motions) waiting to go through the anus or exit. As in Jenny's case, haemorrhoids may be indicated by bright-red blood on the toilet

paper, in streaks on the motions, or in the pan. With large, prolapsed piles blood may actually drip from the back passage. Massive blood loss can result from a pile, even without this dramatic symptom, and a small steady loss can add up.

Inflammatory Bowel Disease (IBD)
In Crohn's disease or ulcerative colitis, or after radiotherapy to the pelvis, small amounts of blood and mucus may be mixed in with the motions. Other causes of inflammation of the colon, for instance infective colitis, may produce a similar picture. The blood is a darker colour as it has travelled down from higher in the bowel.

Rectal Ulcer
These usually occur singly, but are rare.

Meckel's Diverticulum
This is a developmental disorder and consists of a single blind-ended sac coming off the colon near the caecum, and in 60 per cent of cases dark blood shows in the motions. It affects babies and toddlers predominantly, but may be seen at any age up to mid-adulthood. It rarely shows up after the age of 40, and is unlikely to be confused with the usual acquired diverticular disease of middle age onwards.

Affecting Mainly Elderly People
Angiodysplasia
This is a disorder of the veins. Small swellings develop (less than 5 mm across), with thin walls which easily rupture (rather like the venules on the back of an elderly person's hand). This condition affects the right side of the bowel in the majority of cases, and often the person has heart or artery trouble.

Ischaemic Colitis
Atheroma, the silting up of the arteries, cuts the blood supply to the lining of the colon, which may consequently ulcerate and bleed. The sufferer usually shows other symptoms of atheromatous disease, even a heart attack. Most typical is pain on the left side of the abdomen, coming on quickly, tenderness in this area and blood-stained diarrhoea.

Tumour of the Colon
This is the most important of the possible diagnoses. Tumours of the colon come in two basic types:

- Benign
- Cancerous

The first group comprise various kinds of adenoma, and if they have a little stalk they are called polyps. Colon and rectal cancers, the second group, always develop from an adenoma, but most adenomas do not become malignant, nor do they cause any pain. Nevertheless they are better removed.

Carcinoma
Carcinoma of the colon is one of the commonest cancers in the Western world, and also the most responsive to treatment. It arises most frequently in 70 to 80 year olds. Pain low in the abdomen and loss of weight are likely symptoms, together with bleeding from the rectum. The blood will be bright red if the tumour is at the lower end of the colon, but darker and less noticeable if it is near the caecum. The leakage of a small amount of blood from cancer of the caecum is too slight to be visible in the motion but leads to an iron-deficiency anaemia. Diverticular disease in the caecal area can produce the same effect.

Diverticular Disease

Bleeding due to diverticular disease is most likely to become apparent in the passing of a dark-red motion - urgently, as with Jack. The trigger to the bleed may be rubbing by a faecolith - a stony-hard chunk of waste matter - eroding a tiny arteriole at the base of a diverticular sac. Diverticula are especially susceptible to bleeding since they always occur where the colon wall is weakened by the entry point of an artery and vein. There may be a serious loss of blood from this small source.

As with polyps and other tumours, the blood will be bright red and mainly on the surface of the motions if the bleeding point is in the lower part of the bowel. If it is nearer the beginning of the colon the motion may be black and tarry, a condition known as *melaena* (*melas* is Greek for 'black').

When to Take Action

It is important to distinguish a minor matter, with little blood loss, as in Jenny's case, from bleeding with a significant loss, which may result in an emergency. This can be rapid and substantial or develop from slower bleeding that will not stop.

It is difficult to assess how much blood has been lost when it has soaked into clothing or bedding, or even in the pan, so a doctor will check for any serious loss by measuring the pulse rate and blood pressure. A rapid pulse and a low blood pressure mean the loss of a noticeable volume of blood.

The rule of thumb is that if the heart rate exceeds 95 beats a minute, or the systolic blood pressure falls below 100 mmHg, the patient needs admitting to hospital, for safety's sake.

Routine Procedure in Lower Gastrointestinal Haemorrhage
Gastrointestinal haemorrhage means bleeding from the lower gut.
What to expect:
1. Detailed questioning from your doctor about the symptoms, their timing, and other problems, past and present.
2. A general examination, including an external examination of the anus and an examination of the abdomen for lumps, bumps and tender places.
3. A PR (per rectum) examination. The doctor will feel inside the first few inches of the back passage with a gloved, lubricated finger. Piles, colitis and tumours may sometimes be diagnosed this way.
4. Sigmoidoscopy. This is an examination of the rectum and sigmoid colon from the inside using an instrument, a sigmoidoscope, which may be either rigid or flexible. This gives a good chance of spotting the slit-like openings of diverticula and any other abnormalities, for instance a solitary rectal ulcer, which could account for bleeding.
5. A double contrast barium enema which outlines the inside of the rectum and colon. This may be difficult if there is active bleeding.
6. Colonoscopy. This is an internal examination of the whole of the colon through a fibreoptic endoscope.
7. Blood tests for anaemia, which can occur with a small, slow, persistent leakage of blood, not enough to show in the motions. These include tests for haemoglobin level, size of the red corpuscles and iron estimation. The faecal occult blood test checks the motions for blood which may not show up to the naked eye. (*Occult* is Latin for 'hidden').

On the Spot Treatment
If sigmoidoscopy or colonoscopy clearly shows the bleeding point it can be dealt with by electrocoagulation through the endoscope itself. If biopsy (examining samples of tissue), also obtained through the endoscope, shows a bleeding tumour to be a harmless polyp, this may be removed endoscopically with a snare attachment. These procedures avoid the need for open surgery in many cases

Acute Loss of Blood
An adult in reasonable health can lose a pint (approximately half a litre) of blood without noticeable ill effect. If the loss is greater than that, the body reacts to compensate for it. Less blood is sent to the skin and muscles, and

the heart beats faster to maintain a reasonable blood pressure for the vital organs - heart, liver and lungs. The patient will be pale, cold and clammy and will have to lie flat if they are not to faint. Extra plasma is produced to keep up the volume of blood in circulation, but it will carry fewer red corpuscles, leading to anaemia in about 24 to 36 hours. If the bleeding is even more severe and the body's compensatory manoeuvres are ineffective, the dangerous condition of *hypovolaemic shock* supervenes, due to the reduced volume of blood.

Procedure in Major Lower Gastrointestinal Haemorrhage
If bleeding is severe, the following procedures may also be followed:
1. Resuscitation if necessary, with fluid drip, then blood transfusion, for instance in hypovolaemic shock (see above).
2. Obtaining the background story - other symptoms, previous illnesses and how this haemorrhage developed.
3. When the bleeding stops or slackens, a colonoscopy can be performed. Before that the view is obscured by blood, and even a barium enema is unlikely to be useful.
4. Radionuclide scanning can locate the general area of the bleeding.
5. Angiography, tracing the arterial tree, in this, area can pinpoint the source of bleeding.
6. If the bleeding continues or the precise location of its source cannot be found, immediate surgery will be necessary.

Surgery
If surgery is necessary, one of the following procedures will be carried out:
● *Local resection* (*resection* means *cutting out*) of the segment of the colon from which the bleeding is coming.
● *Subtotal colectomy*, that is the removal of a large part of the colon, necessary if the bleeding site has not been identified.
● *Right hemicolectomy*, in which case resection of the whole of the right side of the colon has been performed for bleeding from the caecum, but this operation is rarely used today.

Round-up
Jenny's diagnosis remained one of simple haemorrhoids of the second degree. When she strained, a pile sometimes popped out of the anus, but went back without help. Third-degree piles need pushing back inside the anus, while the fourth-degree type are prolapsed permanently. Jenny's pile bled only slightly, and she was not anaemic. All that she needed was an injection into the pile as an outpatient and a review of the fibre in her diet. It was important to avoid constipation. Her doctor asked her to report

any changes in her bowel habit, but no other treatment was required.

Jack's diagnosis was diverticulosis. He had strict instructions to stop smoking, reduce his alcohol intake and follow the dietician's advice. This included plenty of fruit and vegetables for fibre and vitamin C, and adequate amounts of the other vitamins, especially vitamin B complex. His over-use of alcohol and poor diet had left him vitamin deficient. His doctor was asked to monitor Jack's progress and see him every few months. Jack was not a good attender. Nearly a year later he turned up again at the Guts clinic. He had been brought in with a sharp attack of diverticulitis, and this had so alarmed him that he was - temporarily at any rate - more amenable to modifying his lifestyle.

Anaemia

In diverticulosis or diverticulitis, swollen blood vessels round a diverticulum may easily leak over a long period yet not produce a noticeable change in the motions. Chronic blood loss - either intermittent, or continuous but slight - can result in anaemia. The first indication of anything amiss in bleeding diverticulitis may be the symptoms of anaemia. Anaemia due to loss of blood is always of the iron-deficiency type. This is because the body cannot replace the iron as quickly as it does the other constituents of blood.

Symptoms of Anaemia
- Fatigue without cause
- Lassitude
- Breathlessness on exertion
- Palpitations
- Throbbing head and ears
- Dizziness
- Headache
- Ringing in ears
- Dimness of vision - everything blurred
- Poor sleep
- Tingling or pins and needles in fingers and toes
- Pain in the chest

Signs of Anaemia
- Pale skin
- Pale lips
- Pale palms of the hands
- Fast pulse

- Heart murmurs
- Oedema: swelling due to fluid collecting, for instance in the ankles

Veronica was 47 but she felt as tired after the slightest exertion as though she were 74. When she climbed the hill to the shops she did not have the breath to hold a conversation at the same time, as she had done previously. Her friends remarked how pale she looked and she had palpitations. Both these events frightened her, although the doctor reassured her that the palpitations did not mean that she was in line for a heart attack. Blood and iron tests showed that she had iron-deficiency anaemia, and an occult blood test showed that she was losing blood from somewhere in the digestive tract, higher up the colon than the piles area. A barium enema outlined two rows of diverticula in the descending (left) colon, but she had very few symptoms of diverticular disease - only the occasional cramp or a headache which may have been incidental.

Women such as Veronica who still have monthly periods, and children, are especially susceptible to iron-deficiency anaemia. The treatment is simple and logical - replacement iron tablets when the bleeding stops.

Treatment of Iron-deficiency Anaemia

Ferrous sulphate (one 200-mg tablet twice daily), ferrous gluconate, or ferrous fumarate. Slow-release preparations will help avoid the side-effect of stomach upset. Some people are affected by constipation, others have diarrhoea, in neither case severe. The occasional individual who cannot tolerate iron by mouth because of diarrhoea, vomiting and abdominal pain may take it by injection: this must be done with especial care since excess iron is dangerous.

Veronica, on ferrous fumarate (Fersalal), had an increase in her tendency to constipation, but was able to manage it with a bran-based breakfast cereal (which also contained iron), fruit and a bulk laxative - Fybogel. She had to continue with the iron tablets for six months after her blood was back to normal as shown by her haemoglobin level. She also took care to eat foods which would boost her iron.

Normal Haemoglobin Levels

Women	*11.5-16.5 grams per decalitre*
Men	*13-18.5 grams per decalitre*

The red blood corpuscles are extra small in iron-deficiency anaemia.

Normal Ferritin (Iron) Levels

Women	*8-300 micrograms per litre*
Men	*15-350 micrograms per litre*

Good Sources of Iron in the Diet
- Liver, corned beef
- Beef, mutton
- Eggs
- Pulses, spinach
- Wholemeal wheat
- Oatmeal
- Cocoa, plain chocolate
- Sardines
- Treacle, dried fruit
- Vitamin C aids the absorption of iron

Lack of iron can arise from a high-carbohydrate diet based on white, refined flour, potatoes and fats.

Chapter Five

Irritable Bowel Syndrome

Irritable bowel syndrome and diverticular disease affect a large proportion of the people attending outpatient clinics. This is not surprising, since the symptoms of irritable bowel can all crop up in diverticular disease, and quite a lot of patients have both disorders at once. They both seem to be due to modern living - especially diet - upsetting the bowel muscles.

Fiona, aged 52, had noticed a whole raft of symptoms that had increased in frequency over the two to three years since her husband had died. What she found particularly distressing was the nasty taste in her mouth, with a dry, furred tongue and the fear that her breath smelled bad. Another symptom, harmless in itself, was the change in her bowel habit. She had never been regular, but now she seemed to veer from one inconvenient extreme to the other.

Either she was constipated and had to take a laxative, or she was plagued with diarrhoea. If she treated the diarrhoea with kaolin and morphine, an over-the-counter medicine, she again became constipated. In addition she was embarrassed that her abdomen often made loud, gurgling noises, always at the most inconvenient moment.

She felt uncomfortably overfull after meals, even when she had only eaten a little, and, except when she was lying down, her abdomen felt tight and bloated. At times she had an aching pain low in her abdomen. She felt miserable. Her doctor said she had IBS - irritable bowel syndrome.

IBS usually presents itself in two ways, either:

- Loose motions as the key symptom, with no pain
- Spastic constipation with lower abdominal pain associated with the disturbed bowel function - Fiona had this type

The colon is divided into segments, each with its own muscles. In spastic constipation the muscles of some segments go into a tight spasm, for no apparent reason. This prevents the free flow of the contents of the colon, so the pressure builds up behind each spastic segment, and that causes pain. The muscle spasms may come and go over minutes or clench tightly for as long as an hour at a time.

Diagram 2

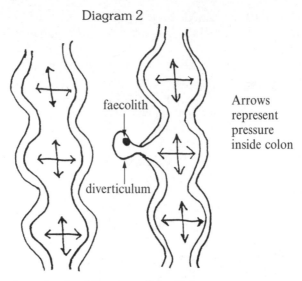

faecolith

diverticulum

Arrows
represent
pressure
inside colon

Longitudinal Section of the Colon

Other possible features of irritable bowel syndrome are:
- Extra sensitivity to changes of pressure in the colon
- Relief, temporarily, on passing a motion
- Abnormal motions: small and rabbity or mixed with slimy mucus
- Feeling of urgency to pass a motion
- Feeling that the bowel is not completely empty (*dyschezia*)
- Burping and farting
- Straining when there is nothing to pass (*tenesmus*)
- 'Indigestion' symptoms - heartburn, waterbrash, nausea and vomiting

Fiona had a variable selection of these symptoms. They came but never went away completely or for long. Statistically, however, most people with irritable bowel syndrome are no longer complaining about it five years later. The symptoms may have died down or the victim has acquired a more philosophical attitude and is not so worried by them. This is little comfort when the discomforts are at their worst.

Pain in IBS

IBS is not usually associated with physical damage to the tissues (unlike the situation in diverticular disease). Pain that is not based on a physical abnormality is called *functional*. This does not mean that it cannot be just as severe and disabling as organic pain.

31

Characteristics of functional pain in IBS:
- You feel dreadful but 'your looks don't pity you' and your doctor can see nothing wrong
- Laboratory tests and investigations prove disappointingly negative - and you feel no better
- The pain occurs every day, over long periods
- The pain starts when you wake or get up but does not disturb your sleep
- Morning nausea, as in pregnancy, is common, and sometimes vomiting
- You are unable to eat anything for hours after vomiting, unlike the usual rapid recovery from throwing up due to a physical cause
- Fatty foods may upset you and appear to be responsible for excess wind: gallstones are often blamed - wrongly - for these symptoms

Symptoms of IBS outside the colon
- nausea and/or vomiting - as above
- difficulty in swallowing (*dysphagia*)
- 'lump in the throat' feeling
- painful periods (*dysmenorrhoea*)
- low back pain
- frequent headaches
- poor, unrefreshing sleep
- TATT - feeling Tired All The Time
- itching everywhere or anywhere
- bad breath and taste in the mouth
- troubles with passing urine:
    frequency - too often
    urgency - cannot wait
    hesitancy - difficult to start
    having to get up in the night (nocturia)
    incomplete emptying of the bladder

If you have some of these symptoms, how can your doctor check that you have irritable bowel syndrome rather than any more serious disorder?
- physical examination including rectal - PR
- sigmoidoscopy - looking inside

If these are both negative and you are under 50 the chances are that you have IBS, but no other colonic problem. If you are over 50, and/or the symptoms have come on quite recently, your doctor may want to do more tests or at least see you again in a few weeks to check progress.

In Fiona's case the sigmoidoscopy had shown a few diverticula in the sigmoid colon, but with no sign of inflammation and no other abnormality.

She had diverticulosis without diverticulitis, but her symptoms were mainly down to irritable colon.

Treatment in IBS
- Peppermint oil or an antispasmodic to calm the digestive system
- Trial of increased fibre in the diet with a bulk laxative, if necessary: this adjustment may be helpful or, as in the case of Fiona, it can make the symptoms worse - especially distension. There is nothing to be gained by persisting in these circumstances

Psychological State

Anyone with symptoms, and specifically suffering from irritable colon, may be suffering from clinical depression (a specific condition, different from just feeling low) or an anxiety state. Either of these will keep any physical-type symptoms going. A'masked' depression is particularly likely: the victim resolutely keeps smiling and feels sure that she or he would be quite all right if the pain or other symptoms (for which no one can find a physical cause) would only let up.

Psychological treatment
The psychological aspect is a most important part of managing irritable bowel syndrome - although the sufferer may be set against the idea. A chance to air one's feelings and sufferings is helpful in itself, with a doctor or therapist who is interested, sympathetic, and clearly accustomed to dealing with these common, but unpleasant symptoms. If the person, perhaps you, is depressed or anxious to the point of illness, deeper psychotherapy and possibly one of the newer antidepressants or anxiolytic medicines can revolutionize how you feel, including all the various features of the syndrome.

Fiona was not clinically depressed - that is, she had not developed a depressive illness - but she appreciated an opportunity to discuss the effect on her life of her symptoms, and to receive support and reassurance.

Alternative Therapies
Hypnosis
Phyllis was in her mid 60s when she developed some of the symptoms of IBS, abdominal pain in particular. She sometimes felt better for a week or two after trying a different medicine, but the improvement never lasted. She had had all the usual tests and investigations, but none of them had thrown up the answer. She was left with a firm diagnosis of irritable bowel syndrome - and a good deal of discomfort. The standard medication

made very little difference. She was understandably fed up and disheartened. As a last resort the doctor suggested a course of hypnosis.

To her surprise, for she was sceptical, Phyllis found that deep relaxation, and the suggestion that her bowel was becoming peaceful too, broke the cycle. She was one of those fortunate people who respond to hypnosis, much as others find wonderful relief from their physical symptoms with alternative therapies.

The Holisic Approach

June was a businesswoman of 45. She had been with the same partner for eight years and came over as intelligent, well-balanced and practical. After a few warning twinges she suffered continuous pain in the lower right area of her abdomen. The diagnosis was subacute appendicitis but when her appendix was removed it appeared perfectly normal. The pain was no better, but now seemed to be worse during her periods. Her womb got the blame and in the end she underwent a hysterectomy - without much improvement.

She continued to be adamant that her problem was entirely physical and would not contemplate it being irritable bowel syndrome, since that includes some nervous involvement. She had never tolerated fatty foods well and often suffered from bloating and was triumphant when an ultrasound examination showed some gallstones. It was a relief to find something concrete to account for her pain, although gallstones, like diverticula, often cause no symptoms. Removal of the stones did not cure the pain or the bloating and it was not surprising that June was depressed.

Now she felt willing even to see a psychiatrist. June needed the holistic approach - to be treated as a person with a mind and emotions as well as a physical body. The treatment began with detailed questioning about her lifestyle.

- Work - an excess
- Home and family circumstances - see below
- Exercise - inadequate
- Diet - irregular: fast-food meals to save time
- Smoking (any is too much)
- Alcohol or other drugs - gin and tonics too often when she was tired
- Stress

June's life was a cauldron of stresses:
- She and her partner were both workaholics, with no time for unwinding
- Their son of seven was bright and adventurous, but was already experimenting with drugs - sniffing glue

- Her father had gone through a triple bypass, and there were frequent alarms when he 'didn't feel so good'
- Her mother, naturally worried, developed a habit of phoning June, including at the office, 'just wanting a chat' but in fact needing time-consuming reassurance

June was neither weak nor neurotic, but suffering from an overload of stress which underlay her irritable bowel syndrome - the painful type. Investigations had not revealed any evidence of diverticular disease, for instance diverticula, which would have been visible during her operations, but the stress which had precipitated the IBS would make her vulnerable to diverticular disease as she got older. An anti-stress programme was required.

Stress-bust
- Reschedule work, delegating wherever possible, fixing an unbreakable limit to the time spent on it
- Build in slots for rest, relaxation and exercise - booked in the diary like other important appointments, and treated with similar respect
- Cigarettes are out - permanently
- Alcohol, caffeine, other drugs and restaurant meals put on hold
- Bland diet (see p. 116), gradually broadened with increasing amounts of fruit and vegetables, cooked initially, raw later. Bananas are a great standby - easy to mash and digest and rich in fibre
- Late nights are out, pro tem, allowing eight hours for sleep
- Holiday booked a few weeks ahead: simple country and sea, self-catering or farmhouse-type. Time to read, walk, listen to music and - most healing of all - getting to know those you love

In June's case she made arrangements to visit her parents regularly and reliably - but not too often. Discussions with the psychiatrist - she did not care for the term *psychotherapy* - helped to relieve the pressure. A couple of joint sessions with Paul, her partner, helped him too. Their sex life took an up-turn. June did not need any psychotropic medication, except for a mild sleeping tablet, temazepam, for two or three nights at the beginning. She learned a few tricks to relax her mind and her abdominal muscles (see p. 106).

Bloating and Wind

In some cases a patient's abdomen may become distended during the day. It is not unusual for a waistline to increase by as many as 4 inches during the day and to feel very uncomfortable. It can be worse after meals, even after eating very little.

There are three problems which seem to be due to excess gas in the abdomen.

Belching
Burping air up is due to air being swallowed. A man downing a pint demonstrates this very well. Some of the swallowed air may travel down the small intestine into the colon.

Flatus
Flatulence is caused by the gas which is passed out through the back passage. It causes bloating before this. The gas consists of hydrogen and carbon dioxide produced by bacterial fermentation of carbohydrates which have not been absorbed. Methane is produced by special methane-forming bacteria, and it is this gas which makes the stools float. The bacteria usually establish themselves in the gut early in the person's life and cause no problems unless the diet contains so much indigestible fibre that they have plenty of the residue to work on.

This presents a puzzle to diverticular disease sufferers. Fibre is good but you can have too much of a good thing. It is a matter of trial and error.

Bloating
More important than swallowed air or gas produced in the gut is an abnormality of motility. The muscles of the colon get out of sync, clenching and relaxing irregularly in the different segments. This allows the colon to fill with air in some parts, stretching to oversize, while muscle contraction in other parts traps the gas. This mechanism has two important effects:
- It encourages the formation of diverticula, and is an important cause of pain and discomfort in diverticulosis even when there is no infection
- It underlies the symptoms of IBS

Tests of gut motility have been devised but are not usually necessary. A bloated, gurgling abdomen tells its own story.

Treatment for Motility Disorders
These are worth a try:
- Peppermint oil (Colpermin)
- Mebeverine (Colofac)
- Dimethicone (Asilone, Deflatine)
- Herbal remedies

Chapter Six

Diverticulitis: The Types

Many are confused about the difference between diverticulosis and diverticulitis. *Itis* at the end of a word is the clue: it always denotes inflammation. Diverticulosis means only that you have some diverticular pockets along the colon. The chances are you may not even know they are there, but you certainly know if you have diverticulitis. It usually comes in sharp attacks and you can be seriously ill.

But it may not be as simple as that. There is a low-grade chronic disorder, with abdominal aching or uncomfortable bloating and irregular bowels at times, which merges into full-scale diverticulitis. Lena's story illustrates this.

Lena was 62 when the illness blew up. She had been troubled with irritable bowel symptoms for as long as she could remember - certainly for the last ten years. They - the family - had a holiday in Spain that year and the oily food had upset Lena. A see-saw between diarrhoea and constipation set in. She had no peace from her bowels, her abdomen never felt comfortable and she had frequent headaches for months, in fact years. At first her doctor prescribed antispasmodics such as Colofac or Colpermin, then antacids, including Gaviscon, and finally Valium or a related medicine to calm her, both in body and mind.

None of them made much difference. It was when her usual doctor was on holiday that she had a particularly bad turn, with colicky pain and feeling sick and feverish. The locum doctor was determined to get to the bottom of Lena's illness, and sent her to the hospital for blood tests and a barium enema. The tests showed mild anaemia and a non-specific hint of inflammation, but the barium X-ray was right on target, revealing a row of diverticula along the left colon. Examination with a sigmoidoscope confirmed these findings. Lena had diverticulosis and was developing the symptoms of diverticulitis.

The doctor prescribed four or five days' bedrest, a liquid diet to take the strain off the colon and a seven- to ten-day course of the antibiotic ciprofloxacin (Ciproxin). Lena did not have the most common side-effect, stomach discomfort; in her case it was dizziness. Luckily she did not need to drive until after the course was over. After her symptoms had subsided, Lena had to remain on a low-residue diet for a month - such stuff as biscuits, yoghurt, bread-and-butter, scrambled egg and sponge cake. This was still to ease the work of the colon.

Following the period of the low-residue diet Lena gradually re-introduced fruit and vegetables, at first cooked, building up to a high-fibre diet. Apart from the barium enema and sigmoidoscopy, Lena's care was in the hands of her family doctor.

Acute Abdomen

This term covers a range of serious abdominal conditions requiring urgent treatment, often surgical. They include:

- Acute appendicitis - the symptoms and signs appear on the right of the body
- Perforated peptic ulcer, or other perforation - including of a diverticulum
- Acute cholecystitis - inflammation of the gall bladder
- Obstruction of the intestine - due to diverticulitis among other disorders
- Ruptured aneurysm - leakage from the main artery from the heart
- Salpingitis - inflamed tubes; other gynaecological problems
- Cancer of the bowel
- Crohn's disease
- Ulcerative colitis
- Kidney infection
- Acute inflammation of Meckel's diverticulum
- Diverticulitis and its complications

Joseph was a businessman of 57, sent into hospital as an emergency patient. His doctor had based a previous diagnosis of diverticular disease on a bunch of abdominal symptoms from the irritable colon range, none of them amounting to anything worse than discomfort. It had seemed like simple diverticulosis until Joseph started experiencing intermittent painful cramps in the lower abdomen, a first indication that he might be developing diverticulitis. Suddenly the colicky pains became extremely severe, and his abdomen showed ridges, marking the position of swollen bowel underneath. He was passing neither motions nor wind.

For a person with diverticulosis, the risk of developing diverticulitis within ten years is 20-25 per cent, with men more vulnerable than women, and more than 95 per cent of them aged over 40. Over a period of 30 years the risk increases to 40 per cent. The likelihood of recurrence after a single episode of acute diverticulitis severe enough to warrant hospitalization is 30-45 per cent. This occurs within five years of the first attack in 90 per cent of cases.

Symptoms
The onset of acute diverticulitis is often marked by the following symptoms:

Pain
This starts with increasingly frequent cramping pains such as Joseph had, usually in the lower left abdomen, but occasionally near the midline. As the inflammation worsens, so does the pain and it becomes continuous. It may be relatively mild and last for a few hours at a time before easing off, or be very severe and go on for days. Passing a motion or doing anything that causes the abdominal muscles to tense up exacerbates the pain. Finally, just shifting the bodily position is trigger enough.

The pain now has two parts:
1. Local pain and tenderness overlying and surrounding the inflamed diverticula
2. Colicky pain in the middle of the abdomen, caused by the muscles of the colon struggling to push the waste matter along a passageway that has been narrowed by a mass of inflammatory material compressing it.

Disrupted Bowels
Inflammation from a diverticulum involving the colon may cause irritation and diarrhoea. On the other hand, usually later on, increasing pressure round the colon can narrow the central passageway, leading to constipation with distressful cramps.

Distension
A distended abdomen may be another effect of blockage.

Mucus
Mucus in or on the motions is a reaction to the inflammation.

Nausea and Vomiting
While unusual in acute diverticulitis, nausea and vomiting may occur in obstruction or if there is extensive peritonitis. *Peritonitis* means inflammation of the membranes lining the abdomen and encasing the organs inside it.

Bleeding
Blood mixed into the motion or streaking the outside is not a common feature in acute diverticulitis. It is more likely in diverticulosis, at the neck of a diverticulum, when a faecolith (hard chunk of waste) has eroded a blood

vessel. Severe bleeding does not occur as part of the acute disease.

Anaemia
Blood depleted in the number of red cells and in haemoglobin because of a slow leak is termed anaemia. There may be no symptoms but fatigue or weakness.

Signs of Acute Diverticulitis
What the doctor looks for:

Tenderness to Pressure
Usually in the left lower abdomen, but occasionally on the right, the tenderness is due to irritation of the peritoneum by inflammation, especially over affected segments of the colon. 'Rebound tenderness' occurs as the pressure is released, and indicates localized peritonitis.

Guarding
The reflex tightening of the muscles over the inflamed parts in response to gentle pressure is called guarding. It can make it difficult to feel the organs underneath.

Rigidity
Strong contraction of the abdominal muscles, producing board-like hardness, may indicate a perforation - the thin wall of a diverticulum having given way, allowing its contents to escape into the peritoneal space of the abdomen.

Bowel Sounds
These are often unusually quiet in diverticulitis, silent in complete obstruction and extra noisy in lesser obstruction, when the colon is struggling actively to move the waste matter along.

Abdominal Mass
In early diverticulitis it is often possible to feel the swollen, tender colon as a hard tube in the abdomen, but as the disease progresses an ill-defined lump or mass of inflamed tissue is all that can be made out. This is either a *phlegmon* or an abscess. It can be felt through the abdominal wall or, in some cases, by an examining finger in the rectum.

Fever
As in acute appendicitis, there is a moderately raised temperature, not often more than 39 degrees C (101 degrees F) unless there is an abscess.

White Cell Count
The white blood cells or *leucocytes* are mobilized when there is an infection to fight. Their increase in number is called *leucocytosis*. The normal white cell count is 4,000-11,000 per microlitre, but in diverticulitis it rises to between 10,000 and 15,000. This helpful reaction is an aid to the diagnosis of infection, and also a defence. Taking a blood sample is a routine procedure when infection is suspected.

Shock
Shock is a serious condition, with collapse of the circulation, which may occur in severe diverticulitis, especially when there is obstruction, perforation or massive blood loss.

Unusual Ways for Diverticulitis to Show

It is important to recognize diverticulitis as soon as possible so as to start the treatment before the illness has got a hold. It can be difficult if it shows up in disguise, for instance with signs and symptoms in unexpected places.

Lucy had the doctors puzzled when she first came in. She was 78 and her main complaints were pain in the left hip and a raised temperature. An X-ray showed a perfectly normal hip joint, but, oddly, a bubble of gas or air lying over it. She was extremely tender in that area. Air is normally found in the colon but not in the skin and muscle round a joint. Infection must have spread from a perforated diverticulum, involving gas-forming bacteria, and tracked down to the neighbourhood of the hip.

Once the situation was assessed, surgical treatment plus high-dose antibiotics, delivered straight into a vein, started Lucy on the road to recovery. Of the rare presentations of diverticular disease, involvement of the hip is the most common. Infection spreading similarly, from a diverticulum, has also been known to affect the scrotum in men, the vagina in women and the bottom in either. The neck, the centre of the chest and the thighs and legs can be sites for the infection to infiltrate. Less bizarre than these is:

Acute Post-operative Diverticulitis
This form of diverticulitis follows a variety of important operations - for example, heart and hip surgery and tracheostomy, an emergency procedure to open up an airway into the windpipe. In two-thirds of cases a perforated diverticulum is involved. The risk factors are:
● Advanced age - 90-plus
● The use of morphine, as is common after an operation, especially in conjunction with a steroid medicine

- Post-operative constipation, a frequent symptom
- Poor blood supply to the colon, particularly its mucous lining

The symptoms and the treatment are the same as for diverticulitis in ordinary circumstances.

Giant Sigmoid Diverticula

These curiosities were first described in 1953, and there have been fewer than 100 cases since. They can either cause no symptoms, as in diverticulosis with normal-sized diverticula, or they may produce the symptoms usual in ordinary acute diverticulitis. The giant diverticula are blown up to their enormous size - several inches across - by the gas formed by certain bacteria. Since they do not usually have any lining membrane, but develop in inflammatory tissues associated with an ordinary diverticulum, there is nothing to prevent their swelling up.

'Young' People with Diverticular Disease

Anyone under 40 with diverticular disease, especially if she is a woman, is in a small minority. This amounts to between 2 and 5 per cent of sufferers, and they are frequently misdiagnosed as having acute appendicitis.

Diverticulitis is usually exceptionally virulent in this younger group, and 66 per cent need an urgent operation when they are first seen, with 77 per cent requiring surgery at some time during their first attack of the disease.

Euan had an attack of diverticulitis when he was 29. He was lucky in that it was relatively mild and although he had to be drip-fed for a week, he did not need immediate surgery. In fact he did not have surgery at all. Against all expectations, Euan has never had another bout of diverticulitis - and the original one was nearly ten years ago. He takes good care of his bowels, making sure, almost entirely with his diet, that he does not get constipated.

The standard recommendation for younger patients with the symptoms of diverticular disease is to have an *elective operation*. That is, without haste at a time which suits them. The operation will be resection of the affected part of the colon.

Immuno-compromised Patients

This group all have impaired immunity systems, because of various disparate conditions:
- Taking steroid medication
- Having chemotherapy or radiotherapy for a tumour
- Diabetes
- Chronically heavy drinking
- Kidney patients on dialysis or after a transplant

Their symptoms are often deceptively mild but they do not respond to medical treatment and nearly all require surgery. This group is increasing rapidly.

'Malignant' Diverticulitis

This has nothing to do with cancer. The term 'malignant' was first used some 20 years ago to describe an especially aggressive form of diverticular disease. It involves several complications and a particular propensity for infection originating in an inflamed diverticulum to extend, not only outside the colon but outside the pelvis. Medicines seldom help in this type of diverticulitis and they present a challenge to the surgeons. Such radical operations as hemicolectomy and total colectomy, removal of half or all the colon respectively, are employed.

These cases are rare, fortunately, and in a recent Swedish study of 392 emergency admissions to hospital for acute diverticulitis, more than 75 per cent were managed without recourse to surgery. This does not accord with the findings by other research workers, and milder cases like Lucy's, do not fit in, either.

Disorders Which May Be Mistaken for Diverticular Disease

Cancer of the Rectum or Colon

It is especially important not to mistake diverticular disease for cancer or vice versa, since the treatment and outlook are so different. The two illnesses can occur together but not as a rule.

	Cancer	Diverticular disease
Previous attacks	rare	frequent
Onset	gradual	can be sudden
Pain - dull, aching	rare	common
Pain - cramps	common	common
Fever	uncommon	common
Bleeding from back passage	common	uncommon
High white cell count	uncommon	common

Susan was one of the few unlucky people who are diagnosed with both. She was 65 and had just retired, regretfully, from a busy job in an export firm when she began having cramps in the pelvic area. It was not the first time she had experienced pain in that part, usually in brief episodes, with a touch of fever and sometimes diarrhoea. In the past her doctor had considered diverticulitis as a possible cause but the problem had never persisted long enough to worry. Now, however, the pain was suddenly much worse and of rather a different character, so he asked his colleagues in the gastro-enterology department of the hospital to arrange some investigations, looking for diverticula.

A barium enema did indeed show a row of the little sacs, parallel with the sigmoid colon - and an abnormal shadow in the colon itself. A sigmoido-scopy confirmed the presence of diverticula and clearly revealed a small tumour within the colon. A biopsy - a sample for testing - showed it to be a carcinoma. It was at a very early stage and there was no sign of any spread. The operation to remove the tumour also included the area of sig-moid colon bearing diverticula, and Susan recovered well. When she came back to the outpatients' clinic she had adjusted to leaving her job - so much had happened since.

As she had been working with them so recently, all her previous collea-gues visited her in hospital and kept in touch afterwards. She told the Registrar who was seeing her for follow-up that she never knew she had so many friends and well-wishers. On her latest visit she was full of excite-ment over an Open University course for which she had enrolled.

In effect, the diverticulitis did her a good turn: it drew attention to her colon before the tumour had done any harm. It may seem odd that so many people seem to succumb to illness after a bereavement or when they retire unwillingly, but in fact it is no mystery. The immune system takes a nose-dive whenever the person suffers a serious loss. Of course it's only temporary, but it can be long enough for an illness to get a start - in Susan's case, bowel cancer. As far as her case was concerned, however, all ended well.

Acute Appendicitis

The signs and symptoms of acute appendicitis are exactly like those of acute diverticulitis, except for one thing - they are on the right of the lower abdomen when the appendix is involved and on the left in diverticu-litis. In a small minority of people the sigmoid colon is extra long and loops across to the right. If a diverticulum in this part is inflamed it can cause real confusion.

Ben appeared to have the classic signs of appendicitis: pain and guard-ing on the right, mild fever, and he vomited just once. At 53 he was older than the average for an acute appendix, but he had no previous history of abdominal problems, which might have indicated diverticular disease. Because of the possible risk of peritonitis or perforation with delay, an emergency *laparotomy* was performed: that is the basic operation of opening the abdomen. The situation was then obvious - a normal appen-dix but acute diverticulitis in a long sigmoid colon.

The surgeon had a choice - to close the wound and rely on vigorous anti-biotic treatment, or to resect the diverticulum-ridden sigmoid colon. In the event, he chose the latter course, judging that it stood the better chance of curing the illness.

Inflammatory Bowel Disease (IBD)
This includes ulcerative colitis and Crohn's disease, which are quite often mistaken for diverticulitis.

Ulcerative Colitis
Although acute diverticulitis often comes on suddenly with severe pain, the symptoms are more dramatic in ulcerative colitis in which the pain is accompanied by bouts of diarrhoea, blood and mucus.

Crohn's Disease
This is trickier to differentiate from diverticulitis: the key features are diar-rhoea, bleeding from the back passage and inflammation round the anus. Bleeding from the back passage is not a definite indication of IBD or can-cer, since it is often caused by harmless polyps without any other symp-toms. Polyarthritis, affecting several joints, and pyoderma gangrenosa, a skin disorder, are common accompaniments of Crohn's disease. Obstruc-tion of the colon due to a stricture (a narrowed section) may arise in Crohn's disease and also diverticulitis, from scarring after several attacks.

Barbara was well into her 60s when she had surgery for diverticular dis-ease, with resection of part of her colon. This should have been the end of her troubles (it was hoped) but her symptoms continued: that is, persistent pain in the lower left abdomen and frequent loose motions. Sigmoido-scopy showed the appearances of Crohn's disease, and she improved with steroids and other treatment for this.

Women's Disorders
Several gynaecological conditions, from ovarian cyst to ectopic preg-nancy to cancer, may be confused with diverticular disease.

Lorna was aged 54. Her symptoms puzzled her doctor at first. She had attacks of pain, fever and tenderness on the left side of her pelvis, and a lump could be felt in the tenderest area. A range of investigations - barium enema, CT scan and ultrasound - showed a round mass attached to the colon. The surgeon decided to carry out a sigmoidoscopy before operat-ing, and found no sign of diverticula.

As a precaution, Lorna's bowel was prepared for surgery with an enema and antibiotics to cover any surgical eventuality. These included cancer involving the colon and requiring resection, diverticulitis with an abscess or phlegmon, or an ovarian cyst. Pelvic inflammatory disease can also mimic diverticulitis, with abdominal pain and fever. Clues to this diagnosis are a vaginal discharge and previous attacks of salpingitis (inflammation of the tubes from the ovaries to the womb). Lorna had an ovarian cyst.

Ischaemic Colitis
This disorder affects elderly people with heart and artery problems. The blood supply to the colon is inadequate because of fatty sludge in the arteries. Some of the symptoms resemble those of diverticulitis: colicky pain low in the abdomen, tenderness and guarding on the left, vomiting and diarrhoea. Examination with a sigmoidoscope or with a contrast medium enema (using diatrizoate rather than barium) may show the characteristic 'thumb-print' sign of little haemorrhages in the lining of the colon. Blood and mucus are passed with the motions.

The treatment is the same as for acute diverticulitis: giving the bowel a partial rest by a liquid diet, fluids delivered into a vein and antibiotics, also given intravenously initially.

Chapter Seven

Complications

It's the complications which cause all the trouble in diverticular disease. Up to a third of those coming into hospital with acute diverticulitis need an operation because of a complication. Unfortunately with each attack the risk of complications increases.

The Complications of Diverticulitis

A sizeable proportion of those developing a complication have had more than one episode of acute diverticulitis. Oddly enough it is the younger patients, the 5 per cent who are under 40, who run the greatest risk of extra problems during their first attack. In fact 90 per cent of them will need surgery - especially the men. The most frequent complications in this group are an abscess in the tissues surrounding the affected segment of the colon, or a perforation. This is the breakdown of the wall of an inflamed diverticulum. A few turn out to have diverticulitis of the caecum, the first part of the large bowel, lying in the right of the abdomen, with the appendix coming off it. Acute appendicitis, because the appendix is also a blind alley, is very like inflammation in a diverticulum, acute diverticulitis.

Phlegmon

This common complication affects 60 per cent of those with diverticulitis who need surgery. It consists of a firm mass or lump of inflammatory tissue at the site of the diverticulitis, with thickening of both the wall of the colon and its surrounding membrane, the mesocolon. It can be felt from the outside through the abdominal wall in a rectal examination, as a tender lump. With the sigmoidoscope it shows up as a bulge or distortion of the colon.

A phlegmon can develop in a matter of hours, and may spread to the nearby organs. The uterus, the bladder and the small intestine may all become involved, leading to a variety of symptoms. Indeed, most of the complications of acute diverticular disease are associated with the presence of a phlegmon.

Urinary symptoms, pain on passing water (*dysuria*) and frequency, are especially likely in men, but they also occur in women who have had a hysterectomy. The symptoms of obstruction also occur frequently as the phlegmon encroaches on the large bowel's space.

Theo started having problems urinating when he was 63. He was always having to find a toilet when previously he could last for hours. It was particularly distressing because now it was quite painful to empty his bladder, and the urine itself produced a burning sensation. A vague ache low down in his pelvis lingered afterwards. Theo, and his doctor, put the problem down to an enlarged prostate, a commonplace development in middle-aged men. As far as he knew, he had nothing wrong with his bowels.

Apart from high blood pressure, which he already knew about, the doctor found nothing abnormal until he carried out a rectal examination. He expected to detect an oversized, but painless prostate gland. As it was, Theo gave a shout of protest. The doctor's probing had touched on a tender mass of tissue, not at the neck of the bladder where the prostate lay, but pressing on and irritating the bladder from outside and to the left. It was then that the doctor asked specifically and Theo admitted that for some years he had suffered occasional bowel upsets. They always cleared up in a few days and he had blamed 'something he'd eaten'. These, of course, could have been mild attacks of diverticulitis, and the tender swelling a phlegmon.

An examination with a sigmoidoscope at the hospital confirmed the presence of a lump arising from the colon, reinforcing the diagnosis of a phlegmon. The possibility of surgery was mooted, but since phlegmons have the propensity to resolve spontaneously and he was afraid an operation and anaesthetic might upset his blood pressure, he chose the medical option. This meant bed-rest, plenty of fluids, a liquid diet to reduce the strain on his colon and intensive antibiotic treatment - given at first into a vein, for immediate effect. Theo recovered satisfactorily, but there is a moderate risk of a recurrence at some time.

Most phlegmons will settle without treatment but antibiotics may speed the process. Surgery may be necessary if a phlegmon is causing intestinal obstruction, or has broken down into an abscess.

Abscess

An abscess is a collection of pus, the debris of a battle between invading germs and the defence system. It may develop at the centre of a phlegmon or by localization - walling off - of an area of infection in the pericolic tissues (*peri-* means surrounding, *colic-* of the colon). Again, men are the unlucky ones: an abscess is twice as common in them, and more common than perforation in either sex. Some doctors have found that over half their diverticulitis patients develop an abscess.

Signs and Symptoms of an Abscess
1. Increasing swelling and tenderness in the left lower quadrant of the abdomen

2. Raised temperature, with spikes of high fever and sometimes chills
3. Guarding or rigidity in the lower abdomen
4. Tender, boggy mass felt by a rectal examination

Site of the Abscess
An abscess frequently starts from a diverticulum in the sigmoid colon and then tracks to other areas:
● Between the layers of the colon wall
● Behind the peritoneum, in the abdomen
● Behind the rectum
● In the groin
● In the hip and buttock regions

Investigations for Suspected Abscess
● Plain X-ray of the abdomen
● Ultrasound scan
● CT (computerized tomography) scan
● Barium enema, given circumspectly to avoid danger of spreading the infection
See also Chapter Eight.

Management
The first medical essential is to drain off the pus, done under the guidance of a CT scan, to stabilize the situation, followed by surgery (see p. 78). Drainage alone is not an adequate treatment since a recurrence is almost inevitable, but an exception may have to be made for the very old and frail for whom an operation might be too risky.

Maisie was 90, with a heartbeat that was all over the place when she developed an abscess from a diverticulum in the rectum. Her bowels had been a worry to her for months if not years, as is common in the very elderly. Now she had pain, as well as difficulty, in passing a motion. In a younger person there would have been a high fever, but her temperature was below normal - also a commonplace among the old when they have an infection. Fortunately Maisie's doctor was sufficiently skilled to recognize the significance of the squashy feel to the painful swelling a few inches inside her back passage. It was an abscess.

Its location made it fairly easy to drain off the pus. Maisie was put on an antibiotic drip and also given nourishment by the intravenous route, and for 48 hours it was touch-and-go. Then she began to improve, and it was judged safer to leave the rest of the cure to nature and the antibiotics, than to subject her to an operation. It has proved to be the right choice.

Perforation

Bursting of an inflamed diverticulum - perforation - is not particularly frequent in acute diverticular disease, amounting to 15 per cent of those needing surgery.

Robert was 67, in the cancer age range. He had been seized out of the blue by agonizing pain low in his abdomen and to the left. He was in hypovolaemic shock and needed resuscitation before anything else. The provisional diagnosis was cancer of the bowel, but an operation revealed perforation of a diverticulum, part of acute diverticulitis, and causing extensive peritonitis. There was no sign of a cancer. After a prolonged recovery period Robert regained his health.

Cancer may be difficult to distinguish from diverticular disease, and since both these diseases crop up frequently, there is no guarantee that an unlucky person cannot have them both. Some cases of perforation cause only a slow leakage of the contents of the diverticulum, causing peritonitis. The symptoms in such cases may be slight, especially in elderly people. The paradox is that with increasing age the symptoms become milder but the risk to life increases.

Fistula

This is a type of perforation in which the disease process erodes a false passage between two organs.

Dr W. H. Cripps in 1888 was the first to describe a *colovesical fistula*, that is, an abnormal passage between the colon and the bladder. He had been amazed to find air (*pneumaturia*) and faeces (faecuria) in the urine of one of his patients. Then he managed to collect 62 more. Since there was no effective treatment, three-quarters of them died - they would not do so today. Cripps believed that the fistulae were caused by 'inflammatory mischief' from something the patient had swallowed.

Colovesical Fistulae

These remain the most common, accounting for 50 per cent of fistulae and occurring in as many as a quarter of victims of acute diverticulitis. Women are unlikely to suffer from this complication unless they have had a hysterectomy, uncovering the bladder. Apart from the characteristic give away symptoms in the urine, there will inevitably be symptoms of urinary infection: low pelvic pain, frequency and burning pain on passing water, and a raised temperature. Sometimes the symptoms are kept at bay by repeated courses of antibiotics, but surgery is the only cure.

Investigations:
1. Cultures to find which bacteria, if any, are living in the urine. They

come out positive in 80 per cent of cases of colovesical fistula, and are a guide in the choice of antibiotic
2. Barium enema to show the presence and position of a fistula. If barium is seen in the bladder that is proof positive of a fistula
3. Cystoscopy, looking inside the bladder with a cystoscope, to reveal, if not the actual entrance to a fistula, the altered appearance of the bladder lining all round it
4. A contrast dye, taken by mouth, that shows up on X-ray, to detect colovesical fistula. The result is positive if it appears in the bladder
5. A CT scan to show air in the bladder

While diverticular disease is the commonest cause of colovesical fistula, this can also arise with cancer, inflammatory bowel disease or after radiotherapy in the area.

Other Fistulae Associated with Diverticulitis
Colocutaneous - from Colon to Skin
This most often crops up after the drainage of a pericolic abscess, or as leakage from a scar after surgery.

Colovaginal
This is another problem that only occurs in women who have had a hysterectomy. The miserable situation of motions soiling and irritating the vagina and surrounding tissues makes surgical repair vital and urgent.

Fistulae may also develop between the colon and the small intestine - *coloenteric*, the uterus - *colouterine*, or one of the ureters (the tubes conveying urine from the kidneys to the bladder) - *coloureteric*. Again, surgical repair is necessary and the only answer.

Intramural Fistulae
These run within the age-thickened walls of the colon emerging in different places. Contrast X-rays demonstrating this are useful in distinguishing diverticulitis from diverticulosis. In the latter there are only the simple outpouchings of the mucous membrane lining the colon.

Obstruction
Sixty-five per cent of cases of blockage of the large bowel are down to diverticular disease. Conversely, 6 per cent of people with diverticulitis who require an operation do so because of obstruction.

One reason for a blockage may be muscular spasm, plus oedema, the fluid swelling associated with inflammation. This may arise in the tissues round an area of acute diverticulitis, a phlegmon or a frank abscess.

Rapidly Developing Acute Obstruction

Due to the inflammation of diverticulitis, this often resolves with vigorous medical manoeuvres as opposed to surgery. These include nasogastric suction - emptying the upper part of the digestive tract via a tube passed down via one nostril, nourishment by a fluid drip into a vein, replacing both food and drink, and antibiotics, also given intravenously.

Slowly Developing Obstruction

This may be due to *stenosis*, a narrowing of the passageway along the colon caused by scar tissue from previous attacks of acute diverticulitis shrinking and tightening. It may also be due to a cancer, but that is easily distinguished by a barium enema. Occasionally a tumour in the pelvis, outside the colon, for instance a fibroid, presses on it, narrowing the channel. Certain medicines slow down the movements of the bowel and so increase the likelihood of obstruction. These include antihistamines, clonidine, opioids like morphine, mild pain-killers and, for some people, iron.

Mary, 60, had consulted her doctor because her abdomen was becoming more and more distended and she was plagued with increasing constipation - except for bouts of what seemed like diarrhoea. The motion was oddly narrow and pencil-like and accompanied by wind and mucus. She tried to account for it all as middle-aged spread, eating too much, or the long-term effect of having had three children. But she was getting steadily worse and frankly uncomfortable. Of course she was afraid she had cancer. The doctor was not sure what the symptoms meant and sent her to the gastroenterology clinic.

There she saw the Senior Registrar. He found her abdomen blown up with gas, and making a hollow sound when he percussed it. There were loud gurgles (*borborygmi*) as the colon struggled to get the motions through the narrowed part. A plain X-ray confirmed the presence of gas in the abdomen and examination with a sigmoidoscope showed the appearance of inflamed diverticula.

The medical regimen for obstruction due to diverticular disease was tried (see above). It was successful in reducing the blockage sufficiently for it to be safe to try a barium enema. This showed that one segment of the colon was very much narrowed: stenosis. The next and final step was an operation to resect this segment. When Mary had recovered from the surgery the dietician reviewed her diet and suggested improvements - basically more bulk and more fibre, and an increase in her fluid intake. She also started a routine involving exercises, for the care of her bowels. Recently she was heard to say that she had not felt so well for years.

Mary must have had numerous attacks of diverticulitis to cause the scarring and stenosis, but she had always blamed her bouts of abdominal pain and wind on her long-term constipation together with the various purges and laxatives she had used.

Bleeding

Approximately 30 per cent of people with diverticula suffer from one or more bouts of bleeding over the years (see Chapter Four). In fact diverticulosis is one of the commonest causes of bleeding from the colon. The thin-walled diverticula bleed freely if they are damaged, for instance by the scratching past of a hard stool or by infection. Serious bleeds can occur from what seem to be negligibly small weak places in the gut. The cause and the site of the bleeding need to be found urgently. 'Massive' bleeding means that so much blood is lost that at least five units are required as replacement during 24 hours.

Jeremy was 58 when he was brought into the accident and emergency department deadly pale and sweating, short of breath, with a weak, rapid pulse and a blood pressure of 70/50. Normal for his age would be 140/80.

The resuscitation programme swung into action straight away. The top priority was to restore an adequate volume of fluid into his circulation, starting with the administration of a salt solution into a vein, with blood products such as packed red cells, fresh frozen plasma and blood platelets, necessary to control clotting. A sample of Jeremy's blood was taken for blood group typing and cross-matching for transfusion. He was asked about his alcohol intake and whether he was taking aspirin or an anti-inflammatory - common causes of bleeding. A large internal pile can also cause a dramatic loss of blood from the back passage. A background of advanced age or aortic valve disease would also have been significant but did not apply to Jeremy.

In his case a sigmoidoscopy revealed diverticulosis, but not the precise source of the bleeding. A radionuclide scan was the next step. This technique detects the approximate source of the bleeding even when the rate is very slow. Continuous slight bleeding can add up to a dangerous loss if it is undetected and unchecked. An angiogram follows the radionuclide scan, and shows the course of the blood vessels in the area found by the scan (see Chapter Eight). In Jeremy's case the bleeding was located at the base of a diverticulum in an area shown by barium enema to have diffuse diverticulosis. The pinpointing of the bleeding point made the operation safer and 99 per cent certain of success.

New technology has revolutionized the management of the complications of diverticular disease. Months of suffering and a high mortality can now be avoided by following an orderly and thorough course of investigation.

Chapter Eight

Tests and Investigations

Frederick Roberts, a distinguished physician of the 1880s, wrote a book on the methods available at that time for obtaining information about the state of the body. They were:

- Inspection - looking at the abdomen: shape, distension
- Palpation - feeling it: lumps, bumps, tenderness and guarding
- Percussion - tapping it to see if it sounded hollow or dull, depending on the presence of gas or air inside
- Succussion - shaking the patient, which might release trapped wind or shift an obstruction. This was an optional extra
- Internal examination of the back passage, penetrating no farther than a finger's reach, unlike today's colonoscopy examinations, which reveal every inch of the colon

Apart from the abdomen itself, observation included 'the countenance'. This could express suffering, anxiety or depression, or show pallor with cold perspiration in a severely ill person. In a debilitated woman the face might show a 'loss of feminine fullness'.

The chief diagnostic aid, however, in the 19th century and earlier, was:
'WAIT AND SEE.'

Diagnosis in the 21st Century

The sufferer's problems and complaints pose a puzzle. Finding out what has gone wrong and why is the equivalent of finding out how a crime was committed and by whom, in police work. DNA fingerprinting and electronic surveillance are among modern aids for the criminologist. For the gastroenterologist there is a whole range of near-magical investigative tools.

Plain X-ray of the Abdomen

This examination, standing and lying on your back, is a useful first step. Gas or air shows as darkness in an X-ray, and there is usually enough in the colon to outline, vaguely, any abnormalities in its lining. The appearances are not specific in the case of diverticulitis, but a pointer to further investigation. Any inflammation, in either the large or small intestine, will cause some distension. If there is obstruction this may be considerable. Occasionally diverticula show up as a row of gas-filled shadows running in the line of the sigmoid colon.

Gas inside the colon, including the pouches of diverticula, is a normal situation, but if it is found outside it is an emergency signal. Infection in a diverticulum or some other organ may have broken through into the general abdomen (the peritoneal space). This is perforation - and emergency surgery is needed.

A phlegmon may show as a dense area in an X-ray, and an abscess may be recognizable from gas within it and sometimes there is a fluid/air level. These, too, are likely to call for an operation, usually after further investigation with a *contrast enema* (see below) or sigmoidoscopy to locate them more accurately.

A random finding in an X-ray may be a faecolith, a small, stony-hard lump of waste matter. While not a part of or a complication of the disorder, it can cause trouble in diverticular disease. If it becomes trapped in a diverticulum it can lead to inflammation, and infection easily sets in. Or a faecolith scraping through the narrow entrance to a diverticulum may damage one of the delicate blood vessels in that area and cause serious bleeding.

When there is abdominal pain, which is often difficult for the sufferer to pinpoint - although he or she is only too aware that it hurts - a chest X-ray can often eliminate the possibility that the pain has originated in the chest. Pleurisy sometimes causes confusion.

One special, but occasional, role for plain X-ray is in a younger patient who has symptoms of diverticular disease, in particular pain, but no diverticula have been identified by the usual ploys of barium enema, CT-scanning or endoscopy (see below for details of these investigations). For the test, the patient takes a drink containing barium. Four days later a plain X-ray is taken and hopefully any diverticula present will be outlined in white.

Contrast Enema

This is a specially prepared X-ray. Until recently a *barium enema* was the standard tool for diagnosing and assessing diverticular disease. To make the colon visible in an X-ray a contrast medium, opaque to X-rays, is incorporated in the enema fluid. The usual substances are barium (first used to locate diverticula in 1914) and *meglumine diatrizoate*, which is water-soluble and less sticky. This is an advantage if there is any reason to suspect peritonitis or perforation. If barium escapes into the peritoneal space it can be disastrous since a mix of barium and motions can light up the most virulent and dangerous peritonitis.

When a patient already has diffuse peritonitis a laparotomy must be performed immediately, without the delay of time-consuming investigations.

In suspected acute diverticulitis without signs of peritonitis, it is usual to wait two or three weeks for the infection to moderate, before having the enema.

Spasm of the muscles of the descending and sigmoid colons (see Diagram 2 p. 11) is one of the symptoms of diverticulitis. It can distort appearances in the X-ray. The details are better and more accurately displayed if the colon is relaxed and fully distended, so a muscle relaxant such as *glucagon* is often given. 'Spot' films are made of any suspicious areas of bowel.

What a Contrast Enema Can Show

- *Warning signs* of developing diverticulum-formation. A 'sawtooth' pattern in the lining of the sigmoid colon presages the onset of diverticulosis.
- *Diverticula.* These look like little balls of white on the film, singly or in rows parallel with the colon, and clustered more heavily in some places. The presence of barium outside the main line of the colon, in the diverticula, is reliable evidence of diverticular disease.
- *An abscess* often appears as an irregular gas shadow in an area of extra density, sometimes compressing nearby organs, for instance the colon itself.
- *'Deformed' diverticular sacs* - that is, having lost their round shape. These are generally considered to indicate the development of diverticulitis in simple diverticulosis. A tiny collection of pus in a patch of inflammation is posited as responsible for the altered shape. Unfortunately it is difficult to be sure of this, since temporary spasm of the muscle may produce a similar X-ray picture. So may sludgy waste matter or scarring from previous inflammation. In diverticulitis the mucous membrane lining the colon and the diverticulum remains unbroken.
- *Fistula formation* - false passages may develop by the spread of infection from a diverticulum from the colon to adjacent organs:
    Colocutaneous, to the skin
    Coloenteric, to the small intestine
    Colovaginal, to the vagina
    Colovesicular, to the bladder
    and also the womb and tubes.
- *Intramural fistula.* In this type the barium can be made out, white and stringy, running down between the layers of the colon wall before re-emerging. It can be several centimetres long, the result of repeated attacks of inflammation. This, and the presence of barium within an abscess, are incontrovertible evidence of diverticulitis.
- *Stenosis or stricture* - a narrowed segment of colon. It can cause constipation because of the slow transit of material through the restricted

part, or lead onto obstruction. The causes include spasm, inflammatory swelling of the tissues, fibrosis (scarring) from previous diverticulitis, or pressure from an abscess, a phlegmon or a tumour.

- *Obstruction.* The causes are the same as for stenosis, only more severe. When obstruction holds up the progress of the motions towards the anus, the result is constipation with blowing out of the abdomen due to trapped gas. In *retrograde obstruction* the enema itself is blocked from running in. This type can be deceptive because it does not produce the usual signs and symptoms of obstruction. Only a sigmoidoscopy or a laparotomy (opening the abdomen) will make the situation clear. With either type of obstruction an operation is usually necessary.
- *Small bowel obstruction* also occurs in a few cases. A longer than usual sigmoid colon may, again, be to blame, by wrapping itself round the small bowel or vice versa. Sometimes the small intestine is narrowed by a mass of the inflammatory tissue of diverticulitis pressing on it.
- *Pericolic mass* - a lump or swelling close to the colon, due to a phlegmon of inflamed tissue or an abscess.
- *Sinus tracts* - blind-ended passages from an area of diverticulitis. They are related to abscesses and if they track along and emerge in another area they become fistulae.
- *Muscle spasm.* The muscle of the colon tightens up in response to the irritation of infection, and this shows as temporary narrowing of the colon in places.
- *Thickened colon wall*, due to thickened muscle. This and various other important muscle abnormalities show up in a contrast enema or CT scan.

Muscle Abnormalities

Whether or not there is inflammation or infection, the most striking abnormality in diverticular disease is in the muscles. The muscle in the wall of the colon is made up of circular and longitudinal layers, which become thicker towards the lower end of the descending colon and thickest of all in the sigmoid colon (see Diagram 2 p. 11). Both muscle layers are abnormally thick in diverticular disease The abnormality in the circular muscle is threefold: there is localized thickening to form circular bands; bands produced by simple infolding of the muscle; and an all-over thickening in addition.

The circular bands are divided into small bundles of muscle fibres (fasciculi), and the different bands can contract independently. A total muscle thickness of 3-5 mm occurs in diverticular disease (and sometimes in Crohn's and ischaemic colitis).

The longitudinal muscle, arranged in lengthways strips (called taeniae), thickens uniformly and develops extra elastin fibres. These form a dense network, preventing the relaxation of the muscle fibres and making the passageway down the colon narrower. The thickened longitudinal muscles pull on the colon, making it shorter. This has the effect of making the mucous lining disproportionately big, so there are redundant folds which readily bulge out between the muscles.

These abnormalities, which are characteristic of diverticular disease, suggest that the fundamental fault lies in the muscles. They produce abnormally high pressures inside the colon added to which they cannot fully relax (see above), bringing about the formation of diverticula in the loose mucous membrane.

Motility Studies

It can be useful to assess the time it takes for material to travel down the digestive canal. Diarrhoea is obviously much too fast, but you cannot judge so easily whether there is abnormal delay. The ploy is to use radioactive 'markers' in a meal, and trace and time their progress through the intestines. Old age and muscle weakness, or more importantly a stricture and partial obstruction, may cause delay. This is one cause of constipation.

An exaggeration of the normal rhythmic contractions of the gut muscle into painful spasms is noticeable in both diverticular disease and irritable colon. The addition of fibre to the diet restores the normal rhythm in diverticular disease but not in irritable colon. Sometimes the operation of *myotomy*, cutting some of the muscles in the gut wall, may be necessary. Without treatment the excessive muscle activity within the colon spreads to involve more and more segments.

Ultrasound

Ultrasonography depends upon sounds, inaudible to us, echoing off organs and structures within the body. It has the advantage of complete safety, and is a speedy way of scanning the whole abdomen. An abscess, for instance, may show up as a poorly echoing area, but the presence of gas in the surrounding bowel may mask this. The same applies to a phlegmon. All in all, ultrasound is not as helpful as other methods for evaluating diverticular disease.

Computed Tomography

This tool, by contrast, is extremely useful, especially when complications arise, and it has the advantage of providing information about the other nearby organs too. Contrast enemas and endoscopies give a picture of details within the colon. CT scans produce X-ray pictures of imaginary slices through the body at 1-cm intervals.

What a CT Scan Reveals
- Thickened muscle
- Phlegmon
- Muscle spasm
- Diverticula
- Abscess
- Fistula

There are differing medical views as to whether CT scans or contrast enemas provide the most accurate information for making a diagnosis.

Paul at 49 had been through three or four attacks of acute diverticulitis. This time was the worst. He had a high, spiking fever, topping 104 degrees F (40 degrees C), and acute pain with an area of tenderness over an ill-defined swelling in the left side of his lower abdomen. He winced with pain when the doctor did a gentle rectal examination. A CT scan showed a mass which included some areas of gas. It was on the left, impinging on the bladder. It also showed a 'rind sign' - the appearance produced by a ring of blood vessels surrounding an abscess - confirming the diagnosis. The situation was discussed with Paul, and a decision made to drain the abscess. Fortunately he did not show signs of peritonitis, which would have made the procedure too dangerous.

CT scanning is not necessary in all cases of acute diverticulitis, which usually resolve with medical treatment. But it is specifically indicated in a condition like Paul's, with signs of an abscess.

Computed Tomographic-guided Percutaneous Drainage
This was the impressive title given to the operation of letting the pus out of Paul's abscess. First he had a barium drink which would outline the colon, distinguishing it from the abscess. A contrast enema would have served the same purpose. For safe drainage of an abscess it must be feasible to reach it from the skin surface without going through the bowel. This was the position in Paul's case. To begin with he was first given several antibiotics to cope with the variety of organisms which might be in the abscess.

A special percutaneous needle (*per-* meaning 'through', *cut* meaning 'skin') was used to aspirate the purulent matter from the abscess, and a tube was inserted to wash out the cavity and drain it completely. Samples were sent to the laboratory so that the culprit germs could be identified and the most appropriate antibiotics used. Paul's pain and fever began rapidly to subside.

Two weeks later, when the situation had stabilized and Paul was feeling almost himself, an operation for resection of the affected segment of colon was carried out. A review of Paul's diet and lifestyle was the top task when he was on the road to recovery.

Endoscopy

Endoscopy is literally the most far-reaching method for examining the parts which are deeply hidden. *Endo-* means 'inside', *-scop* equals 'look', and an endoscope, is basically a viewing tube which is passed into the body via the rectum when large bowel disease is suspected. The magic lies in the fibreoptics, flexible fibres which can convey light through the twists and turns of the large intestine and, in the case of a full colonoscopy, enable the examiner to view the whole of its inside. This requires considerable skill in the operator as well as the remarkable powers of the instrument. In most circumstances a less extensive endoscopy is adequate.

Proctoscopy

A proctoscope is only a few inches long, only reaching as far as the junction between the rectum and the sigmoid colon. It need not be flexible, but gives a useful view of the rectum. Sigmoidoscopes are longer and may either be rigid, with limited viewing, or flexible with a greater range.

Sigmoidoscopy

This is useful for assessing the extent of the disease in diverticulosis or diverticulitis, and even more importantly it allows the doctor to check for any other abnormality in that vulnerable area of the colon. Left-sided abdominal pain may be due to causes other than diverticular disease, for instance Crohn's disease, ischaemic colitis, ulcerative colitis, polyps or cancer. The contrast enema can miss any of these if there are a lot of diverticula to confuse the picture. In cases of stricture - a narrowing of the passageway down the colon - or of complete obstruction, the cause may be visible with the sigmoidoscope.

Radionuclide Scans

This investigation is of especial value when the source of continuing bleeding has not been found by contrast enema or endoscopy. A tiny trickle, as slow as a tenth of a millilitre a minute, can be detected by this method. A short-lived radioactive compound, for example 99mtechnetium, is injected into the bloodstream. It is cleared from the circulation within minutes by the liver and spleen, and after that any radioactivity seen outside these organs indicates a bleeding site. The whole procedure takes less than 15 minutes - useful when there is active bleeding. Since 90 per cent of the radioactive material is gone after seven minutes, this type of scan, although it catches very slight, but continuous blood loss, can miss intermittent bleeding.

To get round this possibility, some of the patient's own red blood cells are radio-labelled (that is, made temporarily radioactive). These are re-injected into his or her bloodstream. They remain visible in the blood for up to two hours which means that bleeding which stops and starts can be picked up in the scan.

Angiography

When there is a positive result from radionuclide scanning, a contrast material is used to trace the course of the arteries supplying the relevant part of the colon - a major procedure. The bleeding point can be identified precisely by the appearance of the contrast material escaping from the blood vessel concerned.

Irene had been losing blood - and her energy - probably for months, and a blood test showed iron-deficiency anaemia. She had been through an epi-sode of pain and disturbed bowels with a mild fever which suggested diver-ticulitis, but this settled. But she still suffered from anaemia and weakness. A sigmoidoscopy confirmed the diagnosis of diverticulitis but a serious hunt for the source of the blood loss, from contrast enema to radionuclide scanning, drew a blank.

The only course was to go back to the drawing board with a full colono-scopy, and make a painstaking, detailed examination of every inch. With heavy, active bleeding, such examination is impossible and an operation to remove the part of the colon thought to be at fault is the only option. In Irene's case the re-examination of the colon bore fruit and a tiny bleeding site was found in the caecum. Diverticulitis of the caecum is rare, and can be confused with appendicitis. Irene's surgeon removed her appendix to prevent further confusion while carrying out a resection of the one diverti-culum that was the source of the bleeding.

A blood transfusion at the time of the operation restored much of what she had lost, and her subsequent recovery - so she said - was like being reborn, with a new body.

Chapter Nine

Treatment Part I: Medical

A positive factor about diverticular disease is that nature does most of the curing for us. All we have to do is lend a helping hand. Even people with acute diverticulitis usually get better without an operation, and medical treatment is exactly what you feel you want when you are ill - sleep, rest in bed away from the day-to-day hassles, light, easily digested meals, and some medicine 'to make you better'.

The other essential ingredients are simply time and patience. It is important to remember that if you rely on nature you must travel at her pace - and, of course, every ill person is different.

Treatment in Different Types of Diverticular Disease

Diverticulosis without Symptoms
If you do not have any symptoms, you will probably find out that you have diverticula quite by chance - from an X-ray for back pain or a hip replacement, or a barium enema.

Patricia fell and broke her hip when she was 76. It was the X-ray of the hip joint, showing a line of gas shadows by the sigmoid colon, that indicated diverticula. It is calculated, anyway, that more than half the over-70s in Britain are likely to have diverticula - most of them, like Patricia, without being aware of it. The little saccules may never cause any trouble, but like the appendix, because they are cul-de-sacs they are more vulnerable to infection than the open areas of the colon. Patricia did not have any symptoms from her diverticulosis, so there was nothing to treat, but it made good sense to take extra good care of her colon.

What Makes a Colon Function Well?
Ideally the colon should be comfortably full of soft, bulky material that its muscles can get a grip on, for the task of massaging it towards the anus. If the contents of the colon are scanty, so that its inside walls are touching each other, it will strain unsuccessfully to push the waste along. That makes the pressure inside the colon increase, with a risk of making the lining membrane bulge out between the muscle, forming diverticula, with the added danger of faeces being forced into them.

The Colon Care Plan

Diet
Check for fibre - pepping it up as necessary. This is the part of the food that is undigested before it reaches the colon and stimulates it to work effectively. That means making sure of three types of food:

1. Fruit, e.g. bananas
2. Vegetables, e.g. spinach
3. Grains and cereals, e.g. oatmeal porridge, wholemeal bread and pasta, brown rice. Psyllium grain can be used as a supplement.

The Government recommendation is five portions of fruit and vegetables every day, and five slices of wholemeal bread. This was not particularly easy for Patricia. She had slipped into an 'old lady' diet of buns, biscuits and cake, milk puddings and packet soup. These are temptingly easy to eat if you have dentures but provide hardly any indigestible residue for the colon to work with. Fats and protein foods are little help in this respect. A high-fibre diet in rats prevents completely their developing diverticula, although normally they share with us a propensity to develop diverticula to the same degree in middle life and later. They also live longer on the fibre diet. We are not rats, but it is an indication that extra fibre is a preventive of diverticula development.

(See p. 116 for a run-down on the fibre in common foods.)

Fluids
It is important to have plenty to drink - of the non-alcoholic varieties. Patricia liked to have several cups of tea through the day and some juice or squash. Tea is better than coffee in excess, and some extra glasses of plain water are beneficial to the kidneys as well as the colon.

Exercise
All exercise tones up the internal muscles, in this case, of the colon, as well as those on view. Exercises specifically for the tummy muscles are good for the figure as well as the colon, and those in the 'colon drill' section are a preventive against constipation. All these exercises are to be found in Chapter Thirteen. Again, it was an effort for Patricia to get into the way of taking more exercise. Her little car, the lazy relaxation of evenings watching television and the labour-saving devices around the home had all conspired, especially since she retired, to allow her to use her muscles less and less. She felt better and healthier even after two weeks of a half-hour daily walk and ten minutes' tummy-toning and general exercise in the morning.

Avoiding Constipation

The three ploys mentioned so far - fibre, fluids and exercise - all help in the battle against constipation. This a bugbear to those like Patricia who, over the years into middle age, have let our fibre intake slip and exercise go by the board. Patricia had lost the habit of a daily motion coming naturally, even with her new routine.

A bulk laxative is the safest and most natural extra help for a reluctant bowel. Patricia chose ispaghula husk (Fybogel) from a choice in this type of laxative. Stimulant laxatives, taken regularly, defeat their own purpose by leading to *cathartic colon* - one that does not any longer respond to the chemical or other triggers.

Diverticular Disease with Irritable Colon Symptoms

The symptoms are identical to those of irritable colon, although the mucous membrane lining is affected differently. The treatment is symptomatic, i.e. directed at the symptoms themselves rather than the underlying cause, and is therefore the same for both disorders.

Eleanor had frequent abdominal symptoms. The main ones were colicky pain, usually relieved temporarily when she passed a motion; loose and hard motions alternating irregularly; and bloating. It had all come on when she was 45, after a tremendously stressful year when her mother had a drawn-out illness and finally died, and her husband, aged 50, was made redundant. He managed to get another job, but at a lower salary. Eleanor was older than the average age of those developing irritable colon, which commonly develops at between 20 and 40, so she was given a barium enema to exclude the possibility of cancer of the bowel. There was no tumour, but a scattering of diverticula showed in the sigmoid area. She was started on the standard treatment.

Management of Irritable Colon Symptoms

- During the diarrhoeal periods, codeine phosphate tablets or loperamide (Imodium) capsules, and cutting out salads and raw fruit until the episode has subsided.
- No large meals, especially of the fatty sort
- Increase of fibre in the diet and the whole anti-constipation regime, when that is the problem
- Mebeverine (Colofac) capsules for painful spasms of the colonic muscles
- Anti-stress counselling and reassurance that the symptoms are not due to a serious disorder

Mild Diverticulitis

Diverticulitis tends to arise in separate attacks. When they are very mild they tend to run into each other, creating an ongoing fluctuant state.

Bob, who was 60, was seldom completely free of abdominal pain, and his abdomen, below the navel, was slightly tender. Although it was hardly noticeable in the day, he often had a low-grade fever in the evenings, and his white cell count was just above normal. His bowels were, as he put it, chancey - one day normal, missing another day and occasionally unexpectedly loose.

The 'Mild' Regime

This can be managed with doctor and outpatient appointments:

1. A few days on a low-residue diet - such foods as yoghurt, plain biscuits and egg custard, plus plenty of fluid.
2. Gentle build-up to a high-fibre diet, and specific exercise - the basic good-for-the-bowel lifestyle.
3. Mebeverine (Colofac) capsules or dicyclomine (Merbentyl) tablets when there are spasms of pain.

Acute Diverticulitis

This is characterized by cramping pain, becoming severe and continuous, high white blood cell count and a moderately raised temperature. Treatments are as follows:

1. Rest for the body, in bed, with plenty of fluids and adequate warmth.
2. Peace for the mind, with no involvement in decisions about anything but one's own current comfort.
3. Rest for the whole digestive system with a liquid diet; or no food by mouth if the symptoms are severe or getting worse (this may mean medical assistance giving nutrition into a vein). These three related items give the colon the best possible chance of healing.
4. When there is nausea and vomiting, or an obstruction is suspected, nasogastric suction may be applied - emptying the stomach by a tube passed in through the nose. The signs would be an increasingly distended abdomen, constipation or the motions coming in narrow strips. There may be spurious diarrhoea, when only liquid motions can get past a blockage.
5. Antibiotics - by vein or by mouth, depending on the severity of the illness.
        Intravenous - e.g. clindamycin (Dalacin),
        metronidazole (Flagyl)
        Oral - e.g. ampicillin, ciprofloxacin (Ciproxin)

A course usually lasts about ten days. There may be side-effects from any of these medicines, usually in the stomach or bowels.

6. Pain-killers. With very severe pain a narcotic analgesic is needed, for example diflunisol (Dolobid) or oxycodone (Oxycontin). Morphine cannot be used in diverticular disease since it sets off a spasm of the bowel and raises the pressure in it.
7. Antispasmodics may be tried for muscle spasm, for example mebeverine (Colofac) or peppermint oil (Colpermin). See below.

Follow-on Treatment

When the acute symptoms have subsided it is still necessary to treat the colon with kid gloves. It will be unable to cope with any but a light, low-residue diet for the first month or two. Slippery elm food makes a warming, nourishing first meal, requiring minimal effort from the digestive system. Dry biscuits, custards, white bread (not new) or toast (not hot), milk products, egg, minced chicken and sieved vegetables are introduced next.

No raw fruit or vegetables should be eaten yet, nor bottled sauces or pickles.

Six to eight weeks after the beginning of the illness, all the fibre-rich foods should be brought back, one by one, until the standard high-fibre diet is achieved.

Exercise, in line with food, is minimal during the acute illness, but breathing exercises are beneficial as soon as the sufferer can sit up. Within three or four weeks muscle strength begins gradually to return and needs gentle encouragement.

Regular checks, at first weekly, then monthly, then three-monthly, monitor progress and form a safety net to catch and cope with any relapse.

Medicines Used in Diverticular Disease

Constipation

A universal problem, especially in diverticular disease - the ideal management is through the diet, increasing both fibre and fluid, and if necessary using the *colon drill* described in Chapter Thirteen. Sadly, quite frequently constipation has become too well established to respond within a reasonable period to this natural method. At least for starters, some extra drug help is required.

Laxatives and purgatives - the term *laxative* implies gentle help with the motions, whereas purges and purgatives refer to a more dynamic effect on the gut. In practice they are all called laxatives since the term *purgative* has a negative, harsh ring. The stimulant laxatives are basically purgatives, and this applies equally to the herbal laxatives.

Stimulant Laxatives

These are also called *contact* laxatives since they act directly on the wall of the large intestine, making the muscles contract.

- Senna tablets - senna is the mildest of the stimulants and is commonly used to pep up the herbal preparations
- Senokot - usual dose: 2-4 tablets at bedtime
- Bisacodyl (Dulcolax) - often used before an operation or X-ray examination to clear the bowel

It may cause cramps or diarrhoea. Usual dose: 5-mg or 10-mg tablets, 1-2 at night, or one 10-mg suppository in the morning.

- Co-danthrusate capsules - DO NOT use these. Contain danthron. Discolour the urine and carry the risk of starting a tumour
- Normax capsules - best avoided. Contain docusate and danthron, a softener and a strong stimulant. Discolour the urine and can make incontinence of either type worse. Best avoided

Bulk-forming Type

These are generally recommended in diverticular disease. They act by absorbing water in the bowel, increasing the volume of faeces and making them soft and easy to pass. They also stimulate peristalsis, the rhythmic contractions of the gut muscles. A disadvantage is their slow action, only beginning to have an effect 12-24 hours after you have taken them. They can also make matters worse if there is any stricture or obstruction and should not be taken on their own at night.

- Ispaghula husk
  Fybogel - 1 sachet in water, 1-3 times daily
  Regulan - 1 sachet in water, 1-3 times daily
  Konsyl - 1 sachet in water, 1-3 times daily
  Isogel - 2 teaspoons in water, with meals, 1-3 times daily.
  Often used following a colostomy.
- Wheat husk
  Trifyba - 1 sachet in water, 1-3 times daily, plus extra water
- Sterculia
  Normacol - 1-2 sachets, 1-2 times daily after meals
- Methylcellulose
  Celevac - 3-6 tablets morning and night, with at
  least 300 ml (half a pint) of water
- Combination tablet - containing bulking agent plus stimulant, ispaghula husk and senna
  Manevac - 5-10 ml (1-2 teaspoons) at night, and if necessary
  before breakfast. In obstinate constipation try 10 ml

(2 teaspoons) every 6 hours, for up to 3 days.
It may cause flatulence, distension or diarrhoea.

Lubricants and Softeners
- Liquid paraffin - lubricates the path of the motions and is not absorbed, so it has no side-effects. It has two disadvantages, however. It prevents the absorption of vitamins A and D, and rarely, if it is accidentally inhaled, can cause pneumonia
- Docusate - softens the motions
  Dioctyl capsules - 1-5 daily in divided doses through the day
  Docusol liquid - up to 50 ml daily in divided doses
- Glycerol suppositories - soften and lubricate the motions, and mildly stimulate the rectum. A 4-mg suppository can be inserted into the back passage when required, and if possible retained for 10-15 minutes, when the desire to pass a motion has developed strongly and the rectum can be emptied

Osmotic Laxatives
These act by attracting water into the bowel by osmosis and literally washing it out.
- Magnesium sulphate (Epsom salts) - taken in water, first thing in the morning
- Lactulose (Duphalac, Lactugal) - 1 sachet or 15 ml (3 teaspoons) twice daily to start with, reducing to once a day. It may cause cramps and flatulence, but seldom to a troublesome degree. It is the safest and best long-term treatment, in chronic constipation
- Polyethylene glycol (Movicol) - 1-3 sachets daily in water. May cause flatulence or nausea
- Lactitol - 1-3 sachets daily in water, either morning or evening in food or drink. It interacts with antacids and may cause bloating, nausea, abdominal discomfort or itching round the back passage

Bowel Preparation
The bowel must be properly empty before surgery, colonoscopy, barium enema or other X-ray.
- Polyethylene glycol (Klean-prep) - 4 sachets
- Sodium acid phosphate (Phospho-Soda) - 1 bottle in half a glass of water, with another glass of water to follow

Medicines which Cause Constipation or Make it Worse
The following should be cut down or avoided altogether when possible if constipation is a problem.

- Narcotic analgesics, e.g. pethidine
- Tricyclic antidepressants, e.g. amitriptyline (Tryptizol), clomipramine (Anafranil)
- Antacids containing aluminium, e.g. Maalox, Gastrocote
- Antispasmodics, e.g. dicyclomine (Merbentyl)
- Tranquillizers, e.g. trifluoperazine (Stelazine)
- Iron preparations, but in some people they cause diarrhoea

Pain

In diverticular disease pain indicates that diverticulosis has given way to diverticulitis. It is a symptom you can't ignore. The severity of the pain and whether it has become continuous gives a measure of the severity of the illness. The only physical means of relief are to lie down in a curved position hugging a heated pad to the lower abdomen, and avoiding unnecessary movement - short-term spasmodic or colicky pain is often the first intimation of diverticular disease.

Antispasmodics
1. Anticholinergics - this class of drugs are effective but frequently have side-effects:

Dry mouth	*Thirst*
Blurred vision	*Dizziness*
Loss of appetite	*Nausea*
Headache	*Difficulty in passing water (dysuria)*
Constipation	

    - Hyoscine (Buscopan) - 2 tablets 4 times daily
    - Dicyclomine (Merbentyl) - 10-mg and 20-mg tablets, depending on need, 3 times daily before *or* after meals
    - Kolanticon - a combination of dicyclomine and the anti-flatulence drug dimethicone in a gel. 10 - 20 ml 3 times daily at 4-hourly intervals
2. Muscle relaxants - these act directly on the muscles of the colon.
    - Alverine citrate (Spasmonal) - 60-mg tablets, 1-3 daily, for the elderly
      Spasmonal forte - 120-mg tablets, 1-3 daily, for other adults
    - Peppermint oil - in the form of:
      Colpermin - 1 or 2 capsules, 3 times a day, 30-60 minutes before meals. Also has a carminative effect - soothing to the lining membrane of the digestive tract.
      Mintec - 1 or 2 capsules, 3 times a day before meals. Also a carminative and may be helpful with distension of the abdomen, discomfort and pain.

- Mebeverine (Colofac) - 200-mg capsules, 1 before meals twice a day
     135-mg tablets, 1 before meals, 3 times day.
- Diazepam (Valium) - 2-mg and 5-mg tablets, 1 twice a day
- Diazepam rectubes - 2.5-, 5- and 10-mg tubes to be inserted rectally, according to need. Diazepam is highly addictive and should not be used for more than two weeks. It has the side-effect of drowsiness

Analgesics
Analgesics are used for pain in general.

In the treatment of mild pain, various over-the-counter proprietary preparations work effectively. Use as directed on the packaging.
- Paracetamol
- Aspirin
- Ibuprofen (Nurofen)

The following are effective in the treatment of moderately severe pain:
- Co-proxamol (Distalgesic) - 2 tablets, 3 or 4 times daily, or in 1-tablet doses for older people. It's a mixture of dextropropoxyphene and paracetamol.
     Interacts with alcohol, tranquillizers and antidepressants.
     Possible side-effects are dizziness, drowsiness, nausea,
     rash and dependence.
- Ibuprofen (Brufen Retard) - 2 800-mg tablets in the early evening, or if in more severe pain: 3 tablets daily in divided doses, always after meals.
     It interacts with warfarin and water tablets.
     Possible side-effects are stomach upset, bleeding in stomach.
- Nefopam (Acupan) - 1 tablet, 3 times daily.
     Nefopam is unsuitable after a heart attack or for people with
     epilepsy. It interacts with antidepressants, anticholinergics.
     Possible side-effects are dry mouth, nausea, dizziness
     and nervousness.

The following are prescribed if pain is severe:
- Oxycodone
     Oxycontin tablets 10, 20 and 40 mg. Dose - 10 mg every
     12 hours to start.
     Oxynorm capsules 5, 10 and 20 mg. Dose - 5 mg every
     4-6 hours to start.
     Interacts with some antidepressants, alcohol, tranquillizers,
     blood pressure medicines, erythromycin.
     Possible side-effects are digestive upset, headache,

dizziness, dry mouth, sweating and itching.
Dependency can develop.

- Pethidine tablets 50 mg -1-3 tablets every 4 hours. Injection: 25-100 mg every 4 hours.

  It interacts with anticholinergics, alcohol, some
  antidepressants and sedatives.
  Possible side-effects are nausea, vomiting, confusion,
  low blood pressure, and dependence. Special care should
  be taken in treating the elderly.

- Pentazocine tablets 25 mg, capsules 50 mg. Dose: 25 - 100 mg 3 - 4-hourly after meals, also as an injection.

  Interacts with narcotics, alcohol and some antidepressants.
  Possible side effects are drowsiness, dizziness and nausea.
  Also as Fortral 25-mg tablets. Dose: 1-4 tablets 3-4-hourly
  after meals.

Note: Morphine, the standard drug for severe pain, cannot be used in diverticular disease, since it sets off spasm in the colonic muscles and increases the pressure inside the colon.

Infection

Antibiotics

These are used to reduce the risk of infection during surgery.

  By mouth for mild and moderate infections:

- Ampicillin (Penbritin)
- Co-trimoxazole (Septrin) - a combination of trimethoprim and sulphamethoxazole
- Metronidazole (Flagyl)
- Ciprofloxacin (Ciproxin)
- Tetracycline (Vibramycin, etc.)
- Erythromycin

Possible side-effects: stomach and bowel upsets; hypersensitivity reactions.

  By injection for severe infections:

- Ampicillin (Penbritin)
- Cephamycin (Mefoxin)
- Ciprofloxacin (Ciproxin)
- Magnapen (ampicillin and flucloxacillin)
- Gentamycin (Genticin, Cidomycin)
- Astreonam (Azactam)
- Trimethoprim (Monotrim)
- Clindamycin (Dalacin)

The main side-effects from antibiotics are stomach and bowel upsets and hypersensitivity reactions (rash, etc.).

Insomnia
Sleeping Tablets (Hypnotics)
- Zopiclone (Zimovane, Zileze) - 3.75- and 7.5- mg tablets. Dose: 1 at night.
    Maximum use - 4 weeks.
    Interactions: alcohol, trimipramine.
    Possible side-effects: metallic taste in mouth, digestive system upset.
- Zaleplon (Sonata) - 5- and 10- mg tablets. Dose: 10 mg at bedtime (5 mg if elderly), and during the night, if unable to sleep, so long as there are four hours, sleep time left.
    Interactions: alcohol, antihistamines, erythromycin and antidepressants.
    Possible side-effects: dizziness, headache, dependence.
- Zolpidem (Stilnoct) - 5- and 10-mg tablets. Dose: 5 mg at night for the elderly, 10 mg for others.
    Possible side-effects: gastric upset, dizziness.
- Temazepam -10- and 20-mg tablets. Dose: 10-15 mg at night if elderly; 20 mg at night for ordinary adult; maximum 60 mg if severe insomnia.
    Interactions: alcohol, sedatives.
    Possible side-effects: day-long drowsiness, confusion, unsteadiness, dependence. (The last is a major danger - DO NOT USE for more than four weeks.)
- Flurazepam (Dalmane) - 15- and 30- mg capsules. Dose: 1 capsule at night, 15 mg for elderly people. Long-acting.
    Possible side-effects: day-long drowsiness, confusion, dependence

Note - the modern hypnotics, zolpidem, zopiclone and zaleplon, provide a more natural quality of sleep and are less prone to cause dependence than the other types, but none should be continued for more than four weeks at a time, maximum.

Depression and Anxiety
Antidepressants
Tricyclic Group
These are no longer widely favoured by the medical profession.
- Amitriptyline (Lentizol) - capsules 25 and 50 mg. Dose: 50-100 mg at night, single dose, for an adult, 25-75 mg daily for an elderly person.

Interaction with MAOI antidepressants.
Anticholinergic side-effects: difficulty passing water, blurred
vision, dry mouth, constipation, palpitations.

- Clomipramine (Anafranil) - 10-, 25- and 50-mg capsules. Dose: 10 mg increasing to 150 mg daily, in divided doses; for the elderly 10 mg increasing to 30 or maximum 75 mg daily.
  Interactions and side-effects as for amitriptyline.
- Trimipramine (Surmontil) - tablets 10 and 25 mg, capsules 50 mg. Dose: adult 50-75 mg in a single dose 2 hours before bedtime, in severe cases increasing to 150-300 mg daily; elderly 10-25 mg 3 times a day.
  Interactions and side-effects as for amitriptyline.

MAOI antidepressants (monoamine oxidase inhibitors)
- Tranylcypromine (Parnate) - 10-mg tablets. Dose: 1 twice daily, increasing to 3 times a day, if necessary.
  Dangerous interactions with tricyclics and various
  other drugs; cheese, liver, meat extracts, wine, etc.
  Side-effects include insomnia, rash, weakness and
  anticholinergic reactions.
- Moclobemide (Manerix) - 150- and 300-mg tablets. Dose: 300 mg in divided doses.
  Interacts with pethidine, most other antidepressants,
  cimetidine, ephedrine, morphine (but not cheese,
  meat extract and wine).
  Possible side-effects: restlessness, insomnia, irritability,
  headache, dry mouth, blurred vision, bowel upset, nausea.

SSRI antidepressants (selective serotonin reuptake inhibitors)
- Citalopram (Cipramil) - 10-, 20- and 40-mg tablets. Dose: 20 mg daily, any time, increasing to 60 mg if necessary - for all adults, including the elderly.
  Interactions: other antidepressants, lithium, major
  tranquillizers.
  Possible side-effects: nausea, sweating, tremor, dry mouth,
  drowsiness.
- Fluoxetine (Prozac) - 20- and 60-mg capsules. Dose: 20 mg daily (for depression).
  Take special care with heart, liver or kidney problems,
  epilepsy and diabetes.
  Interactions: lithium, anti-epileptic drugs, some
  antidepressants.

Possible side-effects: headache, stomach or bowel upset, insomnia, dizziness, anxiety, drowsiness, and allergic reactions - rash, joint pain.

Related types of drug
● Venlafaxine (Efexor XL) - 75- and 150-mg capsules. Dose: 75 mg daily with food, increasing after a fortnight, if necessary.
> *Take special care with heart disease, epilepsy, use of social drugs.*
> *Interactions: most other drugs given for psychological problems.*
> *Possible side-effects: nausea, headache, insomnia, blood pressure variations, rash, impotence, sweating.*
● Mirtazepine (Zispin) - 30-mg tablets. Dose: 30 mg at night. Withdraw slowly 4-6 months after recovery from depression.
> *Interactions: alcohol, MAOI antidepressants, tranquillizers.*
> *Possible side-effects: weight gain, swelling ankles, jaundice, blood disorder leading to dangerous vulnerability to infection (agranulocytosis).*

There are many other antidepressants but these are representative of the various classes.

Anxiolytics (Calming Medicines)
Benzodiazepines
These are addictive and should be used for no longer than 2-4 weeks. They include Valium, Ativan, Librium, Tranxene and Xanax.
● Lorazepam (Ativan) - 1 mg and 2.5 mg. Dose: 1-4 mg daily in divided doses; elderly, 0.5-2 mg daily, divided doses.
> *Possible side-effects: dependence on the drug, and with accumulation, possible confusion, unsteadiness leading to falls,*
especially in seniors. Most likely with Valium, Librium or Tranxene.
Non-benzodiazepine anxiolytics
● Buspirone (Buspar) - 5- and 10-mg tablets. Dose: 5 mg 2 or 3 times a day, increasing if necessary after 2-3 days.
> *There should be medically supervised withdrawal of any benzodiazepine before starting Buspar.*
> *Interactions: MAOI antidepressants.*
> *Possible side-effects: dizziness, headache, feeling of excitement, nausea; rarely - chest pain, confusion.*

Beta-blockers
Beta-blockers are particularly good at dealing with the physical symp-

toms of anxiety such as palpitations, upset stomach or bowels, and tremor. They are also used to control high blood pressure and may cause a feeling of fatigue, or dizziness if the blood pressure is lowered too much.

- Oxprenolol (Trasicor) - 20-, 40- and 80-mg tablets. Dose: 40-80 mg daily in 1 or 2 divided doses.
- Propanolol (Inderal) - 10-, 40- and 80-mg tablets. Dose: 40 mg daily, increasing to twice or 3 times daily as needed.

Antihistamine
- Hydroxyzine (Atarax) - 10- and 25-mg tablets. Dose: 50-100 mg, 4 times daily.
    Interactions: alcohol, tranquillizers and sleeping tablets.
    Possible side-effects: impaired judgement, clumsiness, drowsiness, dry mouth, difficulty passing water, constipation, blurred vision.

Anaemia
Iron Preparations
These should not be taken if there is any sign of obstruction or ulceration or there has been a peptic ulcer in the past. Use only with doctor's advice.

- Ferrous sulphate (Ferrograd, Slow-Fe)
- Ferrous fumarate (Fersaday, Fersamal, Galfer)
- Ferrous gluconate (Ferfolic)
    Interactions: tetracycline, antacids.
    Possible side-effects: dark motions, stomach and bowel upsets.

Chapter Ten

Treatment Part II: Surgical

In most cases of diverticular disease, medical treatment is effective. When there are complications, surgical attention may be necessary. When rest and medication fail to control bleeding, for example, something more must be done. This applies in 10 to 25 per cent of cases.

Bleeding that Cannot Be Controlled by Medical Means

Most episodes of bleeding from the colon settle either spontaneously or with minor medical help, but in 10 to 25 per cent of patients blood loss continues. It need not be an obvious haemorrhage; a continuous seeping away of the valuable fluid also requires surgery. It is of vital importance to locate the place where the blood is coming from as accurately as possible, so that the surgeon can remove the part of the colon that is responsible.

Searching by colonoscopy can be difficult if there is blood in the colon obscuring the view, but sometimes a small bleeding blood vessel can be detected and dealt with on the spot by electrocoagulation. This is a method that can be applied through an endoscope, either a sigmoidoscope or a colonoscope, to seal off a small leak.

Helena was 71. She had lived with diverticulitis for a decade when it became complicated by severe iron-deficiency anaemia. She felt exhausted all the time and was pale and depressed, but taking iron tablets upset her bowels which were troublesome at best. Unfortunately the bleeding was intermittent and although great efforts were made to find the vessel that was leaking, they were unsuccessful. The situation was becoming dangerous.

The consultants, medical and surgical, concerned with Helena's care weighed the pros and cons of various procedures. 'Blind' resection, i.e. cutting out the segment of colon where there are the most diverticula, carries a 33 per cent risk of leaving the bleeding point undiscovered, with further blood loss and a high mortality.

The operations Helena's consultants were considering were:
- Segmental colectomy - just cutting out the segment believed to be affected
- Hemicolectomy - removing half the colon
- Total or subtotal colectomy - resecting practically the whole of the colon

Bleeding diverticulosis is equally likely on the right as on the left side, so hemicolectomy - removing half the colon - involves a 50:50 chance of leaving the wrong side. Total colectomy is four times safer than trying to cut away only the affected segment or the affected side. Any one of a large cluster of diverticula may be responsible for the bleeding, while frequently it is a solitary, out-of-the-way diverticulum which is responsible.

When a part or all of the colon has been cut out it is examined carefully in the hope of identifying the bleeding point. A clot near the entrance to a diverticulum is evidence of bleeding due to diverticulosis in particular.

Whichever operation is chosen, it involves another choice. The cut ends of the colon, above and below the part removed, may be joined together immediately (*primary anastomosis*), while the *secondary* option involves a second operation to do this repair. The latter necessitates making a temporary *colostomy*, an artificial anus at the front of the abdomen, and re-establishing the continuity of the colon later. This is the safer option, particularly if a large amount of colon is removed at the initial operation.

Helena's doctors decided on a subtotal colectomy, because, although they tried doing a further colonoscopy during the surgery, they could not be sure of the exact source of the bleeding. They also chose to delay the joining up of the colon (anastomosis) until Helena had had time to recover from the resection itself, since she was already weakened by the continued loss of blood. It meant several weeks in hospital, but she regained her strength well, especially after a blood transfusion had cracked the anaemia.

Perforation

The bursting of a weak place in the wall of a diverticulum - perforation - allows its contents to spill into the peritoneal space. If this is limited it may be possible to patch and oversew the perforation with a piece of membrane.

Suppurative Peritonitis

This results if pus from the diverticulum involves the peritoneum. The urgent surgical treatment is to fashion a temporary colostomy, drain out the pus and 'wash' the peritoneum. There is then a choice between resecting the offending part of the colon or leaving it to heal with antibiotic cover after washing. The purpose of the colostomy is to divert the contents of the colon from the area surrounding the perforation. It is usually three to six months later before it is safe to close the colostomy and join the colon up. Surgeons are divided over whether resection is absolutely necessary, but the majority feel it safer to get rid of the diseased tissue.

Faecal Peritonitis

This occurs when the peritoneum has been contaminated by the motions in the colon escaping through the perforated diverticulum into the peritoneal space. In this type the infection is more virulent and resection is always necessary. Without resection, there is a more than 70 per cent likelihood of a recurrence, three times the risk after resection.

Abscess

The technique of draining an abscess under computerized tomographic (CT) scan guidance has saved many patients from the dangers of an emergency operation. A planned strategy can be set in motion instead. When the abscess has been drained there is time to assess which type of resection will best suit the individual case, and to carry it out at a time chosen by the sufferer and his or her medical advisers. Simple drainage alone is seldom satisfactory. It is a little better with a temporary colostomy which diverts the contents of the colon from going through the abscess area, with the risk of spreading the infection.

Some abscesses are not accessible to CT scanning, and others just do not resolve after being drained. For these, there are well-tried surgical techniques which can be used. Primary resection has the advantage of removing the diseased colon promptly, so it is no longer a focus for further sepsis, and the anastomosis restores the continuity of the colon straight away. However, the success of this procedure depends on the rest of the colon being healthy. A colostomy from the part of the colon above the abscess site diverts its contents, motions in the making, from the inflamed area round the abscess site. It is an insurance against the abscess recurring or a fistula developing. This means a two-stage operation, the closure of the colostomy being the second part.

Fistula

Colonic fistulae are false passages from the colon into adjacent organs, made by ulcerating infection originally from a diverticulum. They nearly always require surgery.

Colvesical Fistula

Cherry had developed a *colovesical fistula* after a diverticular abscess, which was treated by drainage alone, had spread its infection in a pathway through to the bladder. It meant that when she passed water there were often bubbles of gas from the colon in it and she suffered recurrent bouts of cystitis - inflammation of the bladder. She was constantly taking antibiotics, particularly Septrin.

Fistulae from the colon to the vagina, skin or small intestine seldom heal without an operation, but the worst of the inflammation which led originally to the fistula should have settled with antibiotic treatment, before the surgery can safely be performed. In Cherry's case the pain of the abscess had long subsided, and apart from the specific symptoms she suffered nothing more than mild discomfort from the residual fistula. She kept dredging up excuses not to have the operation until finally the medics stopped pressing it. She was scared.

It was her husband who put his foot down in the end. They were only in their fifties, but he felt their house smelled of faeces and bowel gas.

The operation was a delicate business, involving dissecting the colon free from the bladder with the skill of a cosmetic surgeon. The bladder wall was sewn up with absorbable sutures, and a catheter left in for a week to keep it empty. This was all that was needed in Cherry's case and she wondered why she had not agreed to the procedure years ago.

If there had been active sepsis at the time, Cherry would have needed a two-stage operation, involving a temporary colostomy to divert the motions from the segment where the fistula arose.

Colovesical fistulae are the most common type, occurring most often in men. Next come the colocutaneous type.

Colocutaneous Fistula
A passage from the diverticulum out onto the skin, although it may develop spontaneously, usually arises after a previous operation. There may be leakage from the junction after an anastomosis, or a percutaneous ('through the skin') drainage of an abscess. The affected segment of colon is resected and the track of the fistula curetted (scraped) and packed with antiseptic gauze while it heals. Other fistulae - colovaginal, coloenteric, colouterine, and intramural - require abdominal surgery of the part involved.

Obstruction

When the large bowel is blocked completely, only surgery can help. The cause may be as simple as colonic spasm and fluid swelling (*oedema*) in an area of inflammation surrounding an abscess or phlegmon, or there may be scarring from previous attacks of diverticulitis producing stenosis (narrowing of the passage). Usually a colostomy is made, which in itself relieves the obstruction to some extent, but resection of the affected segment and anastomosis to repair the gap left in the colon, without a colostomy, may be tried. One technique, only likely to be successful if the blockage is not total, involves inserting a wide tube into the rectum and through the repaired colon and washing out and emptying the upper part. At the other extreme a total colectomy - removal of the whole of the colon - is the safest option. This applies particularly when there is doubt about whether the blockage is due to cancer of the bowel.

Resection

Operations available for diverticulitis with an abscess, phlegmon or some cases of obstruction or fistula.

One-stage procedure:
- Primary resection of the diseased part and immediate anastomosis, joining the cut ends of the colon: no colostomy

Two-stage operations:
- Hartmann operation (see below) - the most popular and well-established procedure for patients with septic problems due to diverticular disease
- Sigmoid resection, primary anastomosis and colostomy
- Mikulicz operation (see below)

Three-stage operation:
- Colostomy and drainage, resection, closure of colostomy

One-stage Operation
Monica had suffered from attacks of diverticulitis for 12 years, since she was 50. The latest episode was complicated by the development of an abscess in a sigmoid diverticulum. There was no doubt about the diagnosis - a high, swinging temperature and the presence of a tender bulge in her lower abdomen on the left. A plain X-ray showed a dense shadow in the same area and ultrasound confirmed it. Monica was in good general health, no other parts but her large bowel had any problems, and the abscess was accessible enough for percutaneous drainage.

Because of these positive factors, Monica was one of a minority able to have a one-stage sigmoid resection with primary anastomosis after the drainage. Her recovery was uncomplicated and she was able to leave hospital within two weeks. A course of antibiotics prevented a recurrence of the infection.

The Hartmann Procedure
This well-established, useful operation has been in the surgeon's repertoire since 1923. The Parisian surgeon who gave it its name developed it with cancer of the rectum and sigmoid colon in mind, but nowadays it is most frequently used in diverticular disease with severe sepsis.

The nub of the operation is the removal of the affected segment of colon and the closing off of the stump of rectum. The remaining, cut end of the colon is used to make a colostomy or artificial anus, coming out at the front of the abdomen where it will be convenient to manage. When a colostomy is envisaged it is important for there to be plenty of opportunity for the patient to discuss the procedure and its purpose, and to help choose the exact site of the stoma - the entrance to the colostomy in the abdominal wall.

A specially trained and experienced stoma nurse (UK) or enterostomal therapist (USA), who will be involved after the operation, tells the patient all he or she needs to know at this stage and answers all the questions. Knowing the ropes in advance takes away much of the fear about coping with this strange new bodily plumbing arrangement, and it is reassuring to see the same familiar nurse-therapist after the surgery and to have on-the-spot help through the following weeks. Later the colon will be restored, and the colostomy closed.

Lawrence was one of those who underwent the Hartmann operation. When he was 71, his long-term, grumbling diverticulitis flared up. He developed very severe inflammation of the sigmoid colon, including an abscess full of pus. The abscess was drained and the sigmoid colon resected, leaving a stump of rectum. A drainage tube was left in situ temporarily to prevent any pus from re-accumulating. Two blood tests, a white cell count and an ESR (erythrocyte sedimentation rate) gave indirect information about the current degree of inflammation in the abscess site, and an examination via the rectum of the inside of the stump gave some idea of the progress of healing. A sigmoidoscopy was not possible.

Ten weeks later, helped by ultrasound and CT scans, the surgeon judged that further surgery would now be safe. Lawrence's pelvis was healthy enough for the next stage. This is usually between eight and twelve weeks after the original operation.

The second operation consists of joining the colostomy end of the colon to the rectal stump. This can be tricky, technically. In Lawrence's case the closed-off stump lay in the base of what had been the abscess cavity. This was now healthy, but somewhat scarred. The new end-to-end anastomosis stapling device (EEA) had recently been developed, making the restoration of Lawrence's colon much easier. Even now, however, not all, but between 45 and 88 per cent of these repairs are totally successful the first time. The others require repeat operations, but no one is left with a permanent colostomy unless they are in particularly frail health or choose themselves not to undergo further surgery. These two groups amount to about 30 per cent of those having the Hartmann operation.

No surgery is 100 per cent free of risk and the most dangerous part of the

Hartmann procedure is the first operation. But it is, after all, selected for the most serious and life-threatening complications of diverticular disease. In fact it is invariably the operation of choice when the person's general condition is precarious.

Lawrence came through the second operation without any problems, and now, a year later, is continuing his life without the old symptoms of diverticulitis.

Sigmoid Resection with Primary Anastomosis and Left Transverse Colostomy

This is another of the two-stage programmes, and its name, though complicated, does describe it accurately. Although the ends of the sigmoid colon cut for the resection have been joined, it is still wise to have a temporary colostomy to allow the inflamed parts to rest and heal. A transverse colostomy is one sited in the transverse colon (see Diagram 2 p. 11) The left side is usually chosen since the motions are more formed there and easier to manage. On the right side the motions are still liquid, because the colon has had a shorter time to do its job of absorbing the excess water from its contents. The colostomy remains in place for at least eight weeks, giving the inflammation time to settle and the operation wounds time to heal. It is then closed and the colon repaired.

For a patient in good general condition, this is the best operation for abscess, phlegmon, localized perforation and limited peritonitis. In less fit people and those with the most severe complications, the Hartmann procedure is the better option.

Mikulicz Operation

This is another two-stage operation, used in more complicated cases. In the Mikulicz procedure, the diseased loop of bowel is brought out onto the surface of the skin through a slit cut in the abdominal wall, thereby taking it out of the abdomen where it may cause the infection to spread. This is called *exteriorization*. It is only a temporary measure, however, and the blood supply continues from the circulation to the rest of the colon. The mesocolon (the membrane surrounding the gut) carries the blood vessels and must be long enough to reach the skin surface for this technique to be possible. An opening is made into the loop which now becomes a colostomy.

When the inflammation has subsided, a resection of the diseased sigmoid colon can be carried out, and the cut ends of the colon are joined and returned to the abdomen. This ingenious operation is seldom performed because the membrane may be too short and the bulky stoma can be awkward to manage, even with the nurse-therapist's help.

Three-stage Operation

The stages comprise:

1. Preliminary colostomy and drainage. The colostomy is made in the part of the colon leading towards the diseased part from the caecum. There is then a period for the inflammation to settle, and for preparing the bowel (see below).
2. Resection of the affected area with joining (anastomosis) of the cut ends.
3. Closure of the colostomy with reinstatement of the passageway to the anus. This is usually done six to twelve weeks after the resection, but some surgeons prefer to combine it with Stage 2. In nearly half the cases the third stage is never performed and there is a permanent colostomy.

Better results are obtained with a two-stage operation, so it used more often than the three-stage type. There is also a time factor to consider - the so-called 20-40-60 rule: the one-stage operation involves 20 days in hospital; the two-stage type 40 days; and the three-stage option 60 days. In fact it may be as long as seven months before the sufferer is fully recovered after a three-stager.

Surgery in Right-sided Diverticular Disease

Diverticulitis of the caecum and the colon on the right is rare in the West (though it does account for 70-80 per cent of the cases in Japan). It is possible therefore that it will be misdiagnosed, usually as appendicitis, and the surgeon may only find out the true situation when he or she has begun to operate. Even then it may be difficult to distinguish an inflamed mass of diverticular disease from a cancer.

The options in right-side diverticular disease are resection and primary anastomosis, with removal of the appendix to avoid further confusion, or simple closing of the abdomen and switching to medical treatment. This consists of antibiotics and giving the bowel a rest by a liquid diet or nutrition via a vein.

Myotomy

Rarely, a technique called myotomy may be used. In 1965 surgeon M. Reilly put forward the notion that making longitudinal slits in the longitudinal and circular muscles of the sigmoid colon would relieve spasm and reduce the pressure inside the colon. If the part of the colon affected by diverticular disease is treated, it should ameliorate the symptoms.

One disadvantage is the risk of haemorrhage from damage to the blood vessels running in the muscles, but electrocautery may keep this in check.

The other is that the pressure inside the colon gradually returns to its previous level. This technique has never caught on.

Recurrence of Diverticulitis after Resection for this Disease
This is seldom much of a problem, and it is rare for further medical treatment or surgery to be required. In a study lasting nine years, only 5 per cent developed any symptoms of diverticulitis. Some people get left-sided abdominal pain (not severe) but this may not always be due to diverticular problems.

Elective Operations

'Elective' means 'chosen'. Usually they take place at least eight weeks after an acute attack of diverticulitis, when the worst of the symptoms have come under control, the patient's heart, lung and kidney functions have been monitored and found satisfactory, and there is adequate time for bowel preparation.

Bowel Preparation
Although such conditions as abscess or phlegmon require urgent surgery it is important to prepare the bowels first. A solution of polyethylene glycol is taken by mouth, or can be administered through a *nasogastric* tube - into one nostril and down to the stomach - where it is on the way to the colon. Then three doses of an antibiotic cocktail of neomycin and erythromycin, or three doses of metronidazole (Flagyl) are given by mouth the day before the operation. On the day itself, just before the operation begins, an injection of cefoxitin (Mefoxin), another antibiotic, is given.

Elective resection of the sigmoid colon is very safe and generally trouble-free, while untreated diverticular disease carries a 10 per cent mortality rate - to say nothing of recurrent illness.

Who Should Go for Elective Resection?
Younger than 55 - after a single attack of diverticulitis with any of these:
● Abdominal pain
● Raised temperature
● High white cell count
● Lump or mass in the pelvis
● Symptoms of obstruction - pain, distension, constipation
● Doubt about whether it could be cancer
● Water symptoms
● Contrast material from an enema creeping into the tissues seen by X-ray or CT scan

55 or older- after two episodes of diverticulitis with symptoms from the same list.

Harriet came into the under-55 group. She was 47. She had been through four attacks of diverticulitis with abdominal pain bad enough to make her go to bed, and was anxious to have no more. She was confident that the operation would be straightforward, so she was upset when she developed a wound infection. It soon cleared up, but she realized that even with an elective procedure the ordinary complications of bowel surgery can occur. They are not likely to be serious.

Chapter Eleven

Treatment Part III: Alternative

You may wonder what the difference is between alternative and complementary therapy. In fact they're the same thing. It's a matter of attitude. Some people are very anti conventional medicine and want something they see as 'natural' and are suspicious of modern technology and pharmaceuticals. They want a complete alternative. That means they could miss out on some life-saving treatments.

It seems much more sensible to see this different style of medicine as complementary - to fill in the gaps in conventional medicine, and add a different slant. Western scientific medicine is the ideal choice for some things, especially acute illnesses like appendicitis or heart attack, but is not always successful in the case of long-term problems when none of the drugs seem to work - that's where the alternatives score.

The basic approach of alternative medicine is *holistic*. That is, it looks at the whole person - body, mind, emotions, constitution, personality and lifestyle. There are several different holistic systems to choose from. In Europe homoeopathy and naturopathy are the most frequently used, together with some gentle forms of treatment such as aromatherapy and reflexology. In the USA, traditional Chinese medicine (TCM) and the equally time-hallowed Ayurveda from India are particularly favoured.

Conventional medicine tries to be holistic, but it is focused on diagnosing the disease process and labelling it accurately, then applying specific medical, often pharmaceutical, treatment. A conventional doctor may label his or her patient a schizophrenic or a diabetic - as though the patient was a walking disease process. Prevention of illnesses traditionally comes third in the conventional medical order of priorities, and mainly takes the form of impersonal screening programmes like the cervical smear, legal requirements such as seat-belts, and equally impersonal immunization, mainly for children and those holidaying abroad.

There is a good deal of lip service paid to 'educating the public' - including the captive audience in the schoolroom - about the dangers of unprotected sex and smoking, and the benefits of healthy nutrition and exercise. The hard-pressed general practitioner, with three minutes allotted for each consultation (including prescription), simply has not the time to advise individual patients before they are ill, or those who have a chronic problem. The latter usually have to get by with repeat prescriptions for pain-killers, laxatives or indigestion tablets - or, more likely, buy them over the counter.

A basic aim of complementary therapy is to enhance the sufferer's feeling of well-being, to help him or her to understand and express himself and to achieve his or her potential. This is why the alternative treatments are often non-specific and can be applied to a range of unrelated problems. For example, high blood pressure, insomnia and drug addiction may all benefit from meditation.

Some Advantages of Complementary Medicine

- Adequate time to go into the client's problems in depth and explore his hopes and fears and wishes and the type of therapy he would like, as well as his physical state, family and personal background.
- The therapist is someone chosen by the client, not the 'duty doctor' of the day.
- Because he is paying, personally, for the therapist's help, there is a feeling of commitment on both sides. The client does not want to waste his investment and the practitioner feels pleased that the client has chosen her or him and has sufficient confidence in her from the start, to pay a fee.
- There is a wide choice of different types of therapy to fit the client's personality and needs. Men tend to go for the practical - osteopathy or chiropractic to relieve symptoms that prevent their functioning at full efficiency. Women, by contrast, often choose the milder therapies which relax tensions, counter stress and make one feel good.

The Down Side

- Paying for treatment is a barrier to many people who would benefit from this type of therapy. Around a quarter of family doctors in Britain feel that they should be able to prescribe alternative therapy on the National Health Service (NHS). In fact, very little is available, for instance acupuncture in pain clinics, while mothers-to-be are allowed to choose hypnosis for pain control and unconventional birthing methods, such as water births, in some NHS hospitals.
- Sceptics point out that the reported success of unscientific treatments may be due to the placebo effect. This is the hope-driven improvement in symptoms that occurs whenever a new treatment is introduced. A true placebo effect usually wears off after about three weeks, but this is not always the case with alternative therapies. One reason is the different expectations from this type of treatment - not so much an absence of symptoms, but an understanding of oneself and a way of

building on one's strengths to become a happier, more rounded person.

Whatever the pros and cons, almost 50 per cent of Americans are using complementary therapies each year, and about 25 per cent in the UK.

Elspeth and Harry both opted for alternative or complementary treatment. They had each been through a mild attack of diverticulitis which had more or less subsided with nothing more than rest, and paracetamol to control the slight fever and damp down the abdominal pain. Neither of them had felt completely well since.

Elspeth was 68, a retired civil servant. Her husband had died from a heart attack four or five years earlier, and her daughter was long-since married, so Elspeth had, as she admitted, quite an easy life. That was why it seemed illogical that she should feel exhausted so much of the time since her short bout of diverticulitis. She was not anaemic and she had not taken any antibiotics, so it was not their after-effects. Apparently paracetamol did not count, since otherwise Elspeth was dead against *drugs* and nearly went through the roof when the doctor suggested Prozac.

In the end she followed a friend's recommendation and decided on a course of reflexology. This is an unthreatening, hands-on treatment involving massage of the feet. The therapist was sympathetic and her touch soothing, but the procedure was not entirely non-specific. There is an area on the sole of the foot, under the heel, which is said to be associated with the colon, and this was the focus of the massage. After four 50-minute sessions Elspeth felt relaxed, even content. Gradually her interest in everyday events revived and her energy picked up. She booked up for reflexology once a month, at least for the next six months, to make sure that she did not relapse.

Harry was a 49-year-old salesman, with a job that took him all over the country and included periods of intense stress. He felt he was expected to shoulder an increasingly heavy burden of awkward clients with very little support from headquarters. He felt that overwork had precipitated his brief episode of diverticultis. Although his temperature had returned to normal for a week and his bowels were acting regularly, his nagging abdominal pain was slow to shift and on the same side, the left, his shoulder ached. The X-ray showed a normal joint, but the pain continued.

Harry had gone through all the over-the-counter pain-killers without any improvement, and his doctor had tried him on antispasmodics and amitriptyline, an antidepressant which often helps with pain when nothing else does. Harry felt he needed something with more force to it, but a course of physiotherapy did not help his shoulder and made his abdomen more uncomfortable. Then the doctor suggested something quite different

- acupuncture, which he said often helped in cases of obstinate pain.

The acupuncturist also happened to be a medical doctor, which gave Harry confidence. It was explained to him that the meridian, the channel for the life-force concerned with the large bowel, ran from his hand, up his arm and over his left shoulder, then down to the left lower abdomen. An acupuncture point in his hand was chosen. From the first treatment, Harry's pains abated, and he was glad to hear that there was a reasonable, scientific explanation. Acupuncture induces the production of endorphins, the body's own brand of morphine.

Choosing the Type of Therapy and the Therapist

What is on offer specifically for diverticular problems.

Diverticular Disease in General
Naturopathy
This prescribes switching to a high-fibre diet over six to eight weeks, taking only water and fruit juice if there is pain, then gradually adding semi-solid foods such as mashed banana or pureed vegetables. Brown rice is next included to soften and bulk out the motions and help prevent constipation. Fruit with pips and fibrous fruit and vegetables which may lodge in the diverticula are best avoided.

A whole-food diet and herbal medicines are recommended to support the body's own healing powers.

Western Herbalism
Suggested remedies include garlic to fight infection, slippery elm to soothe the gut, and German chamomile, marshmallow and peppermint to prevent indigestion.

Hydrotherapy
Alternating hot and cold sitz baths or hot and cold compresses to the abdomen aim at reducing inflammation in the colon, but should not be used if you have a weak heart.

Constipation
A host of alternative therapies are often recommended for this fundamental problem in diverticular disease:
- Massage
- Touch therapy
- Acupuncture
- Naturopathy

- Ayurveda
- Homoeopathy
- Western herbalism
- Dietary therapy

Flatulence
This is another common problem in diverticular disease. Recommended are:
- Aromatherapy
- Chinese herbalism
- Western herbalism
- Naturopathy
- Yoga
- Breathing and relaxation therapies
- Dietary therapy

Diarrhoea
- Naturopathy
- Homoeopathy
- Western and Chinese herbalism
- Breathing and relaxation therapies
- Dietary therapy
- Meditation

Irritable bowel symptoms
- Massage
- Reflexology
- Acupuncture
- Qigong
- Yoga
- Homoeopathy
- Hypnotherapy
- Meditation
- Western and Chinese herbalism
- Psychotherapy

The Therapies

Homoeopathy
This is popular in Europe and India but less so in the USA, which has had a long love affair with orthodox medicine. It was a going concern in the

days of Hippocrates, 450 BC, and was rediscovered around 1811 by the German, Dr Samuel Hahnemann.

The Principles
Vitalism - A life-force normally keeps the body healthy. If this is over-whelmed, illness results. Symptoms show that the body is defending itself, and treatment is aimed at giving it a hand.
The Law of Similars - 'Like cures like' - this is the origin of the word 'homo-eopathy' (*hom*- means 'same', and *path*- means 'disease'). Examples are rubbing snow into chilblains or giving pollen for hay fever.
The Law of Potentization - The more a medicine is diluted, the better it works. This applies even when not a single molecule of it is left in any given dose - a stumbling block for sceptics.
The patient's constitution is assessed as well as his or her symptoms, and a unique combination of remedies is employed, combining several at a time chosen specifically for the individual's needs. With such dilute medication there is no danger of side-effects. Homoeopathy has nothing special to offer for straight diverticular disease, but where there are irritable bowel symptoms several homeopathic drugs may be helpful:

- Cantharis for burning abdominal pain
- Nux vomica for wind, bloating and ineffectual urges to pass a motion
- Colchicum for watery motions, griping and nausea

The first consultation can last two hours as the patient's personality and constitutional type are identified and labelled according to the remedy that fits it. Those with gastrointestinal problems are the *lycopodium* type - capable of high achievement, but insecure and intolerant of treatment or of being ill at all.

Ayurveda
Ayurveda is another major, traditional holistic system of medicine - the name is Sanskrit for 'science of life'. It originated in the Indian subconti-nent in about 2,500 BC and is increasingly popular today, particularly in the USA.

The Principles
The vital forces are divided into three *doshas* - *vata*, *pitta* - and *kapha*, each associated with a particular character and body type. Vata is the dosha based in the colon. When it is out of order the illness is likely to flare up in the early morning, but to respond to calming medicines at night.

Foods which calm symptoms - moist, warming foods pacify vata: casseroles, vegetable soup, cooked carrots.

Foods which make the symptoms worse - anything raw, bitter or pungent.

Ayurveda is not specifically recommended for diverticular disease, but an ayurvedic prescription for constipation is the laxative, *triphala* powder; a fruit and vegetable diet with wholemeal cereals and bran; and Yoga exercises. The powerful cleansing routines, such as *panchakarma*, can precipitate rather than cure disturbances of the bowel in diverticular disease, but a warm milk drink with ginger, cinnamon or cardamom before bed puts the colon as well as the mind to rest. Most ayurvedic prescriptions contain at least ten different herbs, and traditionally the practitioner repeats a mantra as he prepares the mixture.

Naturopathy

Nature cure, Natural medicine, and, as it came to be called, Naturopathy is rooted in the mists of history. It seems always to have been with us but it was 'discovered', brushed off and organized in the late 19th century. The name was coined in 1895 by Dr John Scheel of New York, but by that time there was already a fashion for natural remedies. A few years into the 20th century, John Kellogg of breakfast cereal fame used the term for the treatment in his sanatorium.

The Principles

The guiding principle is that the body has the power to heal itself, and needs only a little help. This concept of a vital force also runs through homoeopathy, ayurveda and Traditional Chinese Medicine (TCM). Naturopaths believe that illness is caused by an unhealthy lifestyle overwhelming the body's best efforts. Harmful factors are lack of sleep and fresh air, faulty diet, emotional or physical stress - and a negative outlook. A plain diet, rich in organic foods, and a balance of regular exercise, rest and sleep and the avoidance of stress are obviously beneficial rules for living which are recommended.

Naturopathic Remedies

- Herbal medicines, mineral and vitamin supplements geared to supporting nature
- Yoga
- Massage
- Hydrotherapy
- Osteopathy

The first consultation is likely to last about an hour, but later sessions last

20 to 40 minutes. The number needed ranges from 4 to 30. Fasting for a few days may arise in the course of the treatment, but otherwise none of it is unpleasant.

Hydrotherapy

Water has always fascinated man - and woman and child. Why else are seaside holidays so popular? The Greeks believed that water contained the secret of health, a vital essence. The Romans built sophisticated bath houses, while we have pools in every moderate-sized town, and saunas and jacuzzis in many homes. Turkish baths have been long established, and on a small scale there are footbaths for aching feet, and hot compresses and ice-packs for pain.

Hot and cold sitz baths and compresses for reducing inflammation in areas of diverticular disease have already been mentioned. The general effect of dry heat or steam heat (Turkish bath) is said to draw impurities out of the body in the sweat.

Traditional Chinese Medicine (TCM)

This ancient holistic system of healing is geared to the individual's problems or just his or her wish for well-being, rather than diseases with labels. From the 16th century Western medicine began to push TCM aside but in 1949 the People's Republic reversed the trend and now both kinds of medicine co-exist in China.

The traditional type includes a variety of treatments: acupuncture, qigong, dietary and exercise regimes and, most importantly, Chinese herbalism.

The Principles

- The body is an integrated whole and a change in one part, however small, affects all the others.
- Yin and yang are opposing but complementary forces and good health depends on a balance between them.
- Yin relates to the shady side of a mountain, the moon, femininity, cold, earth, deficiency - and apart from the bowels only the outside of the body.
- Yang is the sunny side, masculinity, warmth, plenty and the vital internal organs. heart, lungs and liver.
- Meridians are channels for qi, or life energy, which run all over the body. Acupuncture points are sited in the line of the meridians and connect to various organs.
- The Five Elements which make up everything in the universe, including the human body, are Fire, Wood, Metal, Earth and Water. The colon

is ascribed to the element Metal, which is associated with autumn, grief, and pungent flavours.

Acupuncture, qigong and herbalism are the aspects of TCM commonly used in Western disorders such as diverticular disease, but there have been some worrying reports about ill-effects from Chinese herbs, particularly affecting the kidneys. These may have been due to cheaper substitutes replacing expensive ingredients in the original, multi-herb recipes. It is important to use a reputable supplier. With the large number of herbs used in each prescription, standardization is impractical.

Acupuncture

This is a method for tapping into the network of meridians carrying the life force. Specific entry points (they number 365) serve different organs. The method involves the insertion of long, very fine needles into selected acupoints which may be nowhere near the part of the body giving trouble. When they are in place, the needles are twisted. This may cause a feeling of tugging or numbness, but does not hurt, nor is there usually any bleeding. Nowadays an electric current is sometimes used as a stimulus instead of the twisting.

Acupuncture is used particularly to relieve pain, and among the Chinese is employed as an anaesthetic in surgery. Its main uses, apart from pain relief, include:

Arthritis, fibrositis and rheumatism	Migraine, nausea
Asthma and hay fever	High blood pressure
Addictions	Digestive system disorders
Depression and anxiety	Women's health

This disparate list is typical of alternative therapies, which are aimed at improving general well-being rather than the relief of specific disorders.

Moxibustion - this involves burning the herb, moxa, in cones placed over the acupoints as another way of stimulating them. The object is to harmonize the body by influencing the flow of qi.

Auricular acupuncture - the ear, in Chinese medical theory, carries more than 120 acupoints. These are arranged in relation to the body as though the ear were a foetus upside-down. The lobe represents the head, the rim the backbone and the middle ear the organs of the abdomen. Tiny needles or finger pressure is used to stimulate the acupuncture sites.

Acupressure - in acupressure a finger rather than a needle is used as a stimulus at the acupuncture points.

Shiatsu - the Japanese version of acupuncture. The life energy is called ki instead of qi. Treatment is said to relieve muscle tension and induce a feeling of peace and relaxation.

Precautions with Acupuncture
Check that the practitioner uses disposable needles or autoclaves them because of the danger of infection.

Miss out on this treatment if you are pregnant or might be, except during labour itself.

Avoid alcohol, big meals, hot baths or showers or strenuous exercise immediately before or after a session.

Qigong
The word means 'energy work'. It is an ancient system of movement, breathing techniques and meditation. It is said to be good for the circulation, not of the blood, but of qi. It is suitable for people of all ages, and was used on the banks of the Yellow River 4,000 years ago to ward off arthritis, but it is reputed to improve the function of all parts of the body.

T'ai Chi
This a gentle movement therapy, used by Taoist monks in the 13th century. It may be performed by young and elderly people in particular, one-to-one or in groups of up to 30. It brings bodily relaxation and secondary psychological calm if practised daily.

Healing
The cure of disease or disability by religious ritual or magic has been known since time immemorial. The laying on of hands was practised by the priests of ancient Egypt, was reported in the New Testament, and has continued with shrines and relics down to healing services in today's Christian churches - and individual healers.

Spiritualists - claim that entities from the spirit world - sometimes the ghosts of loved ones - take over the healer's body and can perform miraculous cures. He or she is the channel, not the possessor of special powers.

Reiki - This Japanese type of spiritual healing, based in Tibetan Buddhism, is claimed to operate at an atomic level. Reiki energy travels through the practitioner's hands into the client's body and tunes up his or her spiritual and etheric life. Adherents recommend it for all physical, mental and emotional disorders.

Therapeutic Touch (TT) - In this form of healing, the healer holds his or her hands over the painful or troublesome area, and concentrates. There is often no actual contact.

Healers often bring comfort when pain or other symptoms have become wearisome.

Yoga

This system of gentle physical exercises was developed as a preparation for spiritual growth. Many people find it pleasant and relaxing and it is used for a host of general problems from fatigue to asthma to colonic disorder. It is meant to control all aspects of the subject's life. Yoga classes are readily available and daily practice is advised.

Ann was 56. She had suffered since she was 35 from irritable colon symptoms plus episodes of mild abdominal pain and a slight fever, possibly down to diverticulitis. These were getting worse, and she also suffered from stress-related migraine. Ann was not standing up well to the extra strains that are common in the decade 50 to 60, in her case the death of her father, her son's marriage to a girl she did not like, and her husband's high blood pressure.

It was at this point that Ann's neighbour, a widow, started yoga classes and invited her to come along too. Every morning now, the two friends both do 45 minutes' yoga, starting with breathing exercises, then movement and holding particular postures and finally the ploys for relaxation. They still attend the weekly classes.

Ann's colonic discomfort is hardly noticeable nowadays, and she has not had a migraine for months.

There are several complementary therapies involving manipulation, but they contain nothing very relevant to diverticular disease.

Chiropractic

The word actually means *manipulation* - 'done with the hands' and it was developed in the 1890s. The principle is that a maladjustment in the bones of the spine will affect the whole body through its link with the brain. Treatment by re-positioning the bones can put this right, straightaway, curing a variety of ills including deafness. It is undoubtedly helpful in neck and spine disorders and sciatica, but may cause harm in osteoporosis, infection, tumour and circulatory problems.

Osteopathy

The organs of the body, including the colon, are supported and protected by bones and muscles. If these are properly aligned and working smoothly, other parts of the body, including the gastrointestinal system, will also function well.

Osteopaths use massage and manipulation to free up the joints and improve mobility. They are regarded as doctors in the United States, but only a third of British GPs would refer their patients to an osteopath rather than a physiotherapist and few would suggest osteopathy for diverticular disease.

Aromatherapy
Cultures from ancient Egypt to present-day France have used aromatherapy, and it has become increasingly popular throughout the West. Essential oils from all parts of the plants are believed to have healing properties, and their scents to affect libido, mood, metabolism and stress levels. Massage using these oils is used to alleviate pain, muscle spasm and digestive problems.

- Rosemary is analgesic and also a stimulant
- Sandalwood is a sedative
- Peppermint oil used in this way is as soothing to the stomach and gut as it is when taken by mouth
- Clary sage and German chamomile oils relieve flatulence

A full body massage takes one hour.

Reflexology
Foot massage originated in China 5,000 years ago and was also practised in ancient Egypt, but in 1915 it was put on the map by Dr William Fitzgerald. He worked out a system of zones. Different parts of the body are represented on the soles of the feet, and treatment consists of pressure and massage over the appropriate zone. See page 88.
Complementary therapies will not staunch a haemorrhage or drain an abscess, but in cases of persistent pain with attendant anxiety and depression, they may give the sufferer some comfort. There is also the feeling that there is something he can do to help himself, with the ongoing support of the therapist.

Chapter Twelve

Herbal Treatment

Herbalism means tapping into the remarkable properties of plants, using them to alleviate illness and other physical problems, and to enhance well-being. Like conventional medicines, no matter what enthusiasts claim, they can have side-effects or interact with other treatments. Homeopathic remedies do not have side-effects, because they are so dilute.

Like other specialist subjects, herbalism uses many words which are not in everyday use. To make the descriptions of the various herbs understandable here is a list of the commonest terms.

Mini-glossary

Adaptogen	A herb that helps you adjust to stress and other changes.
Example:	**Siberian Ginseng.**
Alterative	Corrects disordered working, for instance of the colon - spasm, constipation, looseness.
Examples:	**Parsley, yellow dock.**
Anti-inflammatory	Soothes inflammation, as in diverticulitis.
Examples:	**Willow, cabbage, camomile.**
Bitters	Stimulate appetite, promote digestion.
Examples:	**Camomile, dandelion, dock.**
Carminative	Reduces flatulence and indigestion.
Examples:	**Peppermint, fennel, cinnamon.**
Demulcent	Soothes irritation in the colon and the rest of the digestive system.
Examples:	**Marshmallow, comfrey, honey.**
Digestive	Promotes good digestion.
Examples:	**Camomile, ginger, oats, rosemary.**
Digestive tonic	To improve digestion and appetite.
Examples:	**Rosemary, camomile.**
Febrifuge	Reduces fever.
Examples:	**Yarrow, camomile, sage.**
Hepatic	Particularly good for the liver.
Examples:	**Dandelion, turmeric, thyme, rosemary.**

Iron provider	For blood loss, anaemia.
Examples:	**Nettle, dock.**
Laxative	For constipation.
Examples:	**Dock, dandelion root, senna.**
Nerve tonic	Helps with anxiety, nervousness and lack of energy.
Examples:	**Linden, St John's wort, lemon balm.**
Nervine	Relieves depression and anxiety.
Examples:	**Camomile, St John's wort, lemon balm.**
Relaxant	Relaxes mind, muscles and gut.
Example:	**Camomile.**
Restorative	To build up your strength during convalescence.
Sedative	Makes you feel calm, maybe slightly drowsy.
Examples:	**Camomile, linden, clove.**
Stimulant	Brightens you up, increases energy.
Examples:	**Cayenne, coffee, ginseng.**
Tonic	Improves appetite and general strength.
Examples:	**Sage, verbena.**

Preparations:
- *Infusion*: herbal tea.
- *Decoction*: medicine made from the woody parts of the plant.
- *Tincture*: solution in alcohol, vinegar or glycerine.

Historical Background

People have used plants for food and medical purposes for as long as there have been records - and no doubt before that.

1600 BC Egypt: papyri mention juniper, fennel and thyme as medicaments. Cloves of garlic were found in Tutankhamen's tomb.

1000 BC China: the *Yellow Emperor's Book of Internal Medicine* lists herbal remedies.

800 BC India: Ayurveda describes herbs used to 'restore health and equilibrium' but the system had been in use since 2500 BC.

400 BC Greece: Hippocrates recommends camomile, garlic, cinnamon and rosemary.

100 AD Roman Empire: Dioscorides, a well-travelled army doctor, wrote his *Materia Medica*, a comprehensive herbal.

150 AD Italy, Greece and Turkey: Galen published his herbal, *De Simplicibus* (a 'simple' is a plant medicine).

1000 Persia: Avicenna wrote his *Canon*, a complete medical textbook, including herbal remedies.

1500 Switzerland: Paracelsus introduced 'the doctrine of signatures' - the theory that plants showed by their appearance what illnesses they would benefit, for example yellow plants could cure jaundice.

1597 England: John Gerard produced his *Herball* - he too believed in the signatures theory.

1649 England: Nicholas Culpeper's *Physicall Directory* came out - generally known as *Culpeper's Herbal*.

1800 America: Samuel Thompson wrote on native American folklore, including the use of herbs.

1930 England: Dr Edward Bach introduced his Flower Remedies, particularly aimed at treating unhappy states of mind.

1949 The People's Republic of China re-introduced by law traditional Chinese medicine, including the herbal remedies. Many of the time-hallowed, historical herbal medicines are still in use today.

Herbs Used in Diverticular Disease

Aloe Vera
Laxative, digestive.
   Leaf as tea or tincture, or the juice may be used.
   Uses: For constipation (the Romans used it to promote
                  the healing of wounds).
   Side-effects: Griping, vomiting. Unsuitable in pregnancy or
                  breastfeeding.

Angelica
Carminative, tonic.
   Seeds are chewed or medicine prepared.
   Uses: Flatulence especially, also colic, poor appetite. Native
                  Americans use it for pain - as a compress on the
                  opposite side.
   Side-effects: Gastrointestinal disturbance. Unsuitable in pregnancy.

Burdock
Laxative, carminative.
   Root and seeds are used.
   Uses: Chronic constipation, indigestion.
   Side-effects: Sometimes worsening of the original symptoms. Not
                  for use in pregnancy.

Camomile
Relaxant, sedative, antispasmodic, anti-inflammatory, bitter, digestive, febrifuge, nervine.

Parts of the plant as tea.

Uses:	All types of stress, physical and mental, diverticular disease - all stages.
Side-effects:	Nausea, rash.

Cayenne Pepper
Digestive, tonic, stimulant.

Seeds are used. Popularized by Samuel Thompson around 1800.

Uses:	Flatulence, bloating; loss of appetite in convalescence and in the elderly.
Side-effects:	Indigestion.

Cinnamon
Antispasmodic, digestive, stimulant, carminative.

Bark is used.

Uses:	Wind and griping, diarrhoea, irritable bowel symptoms. Used in India for indigestion and was contained in the original British digestive biscuits. The Chinese used it to cure cold feet, and the Egyptians put it in perfume.
Side-effects:	Rumbling tummy, not advised in pregnancy

Comfrey
Anti-inflammatory, demulcent.

Leaves in tea or tincture.

Uses:	Diverticulitis, hiatus hernia; also switches off breast milk.
Side-effects:	Turning off milk if that is not wanted.

Dandelion
Laxative, bitter, hepatic, restorative.

Leaves, root and flowers.

Uses:	Chronic constipation, used as a coffee substitute, especially with chicory.
Side-effects:	Griping.

Dock
Gentle laxative, alternative, source of iron, bitter.

Leaves.

Uses:	Mild constipation, anaemia, and as an application in insect bites and stings and nettle stings. Were put into shoes by Romans and others for walking long distances.
Side-effects:	None described.

Fennel
Antispasmodic, demulcent, carminative.

Leaves, stalk.

Uses:	Feeling too full, wind, irritable bowel symptoms. Chewed by the ancient Greeks and in Europe in the Middle Ages to suppress hunger during religious fasts.
Side-effects:	Must not be used in pregnancy except in cooking.

Ginger
Carminative, digestive, anti-diarrhoeal, anti-nauseant.

Hot ginger tea or chewing crystallized ginger.

Uses:	To damp down nausea, or, taken after a meal, to settle the digestive system, including the colon. The early Greeks and Indians used it, and the Chinese 'to cleanse their aura'.
Side-effects:	Negligible.

Hawthorn
Carminative, restorative.

Flowers, berries.

Uses:	Flatulence, fullness, colic. The Chinese use it for diarrhoea. There is a superstition that it foreshadows a death if it is brought indoors, but it brings good luck at weddings.
Side-effects:	Lowers blood pressure and interacts with some heart drugs. Not to be used when there are heart or blood pressure problems.

Marshmallow
Demulcent, nutritive.

Leaves may be eaten cooked like spinach, or the flowers in a salad; the seeds are used in traditional Chinese medicine.

Uses:	Soothing the digestive system, nourishing.
Side-effects:	None described.

Mugwort
Digestive, febrifuge.
Leaves may be chewed or put in your shoes.

Uses: Relief of indigestion and cramps, fever, headache and depression. Used in the shoes to revive tired feet since Roman times. In 1656 William Coles, in *The Art of Simpling*, said a foot soldier could walk 40 miles a day using mugwort. Can also be smoked - known as 'poor man's tobacco'.

Side-effects: None mentioned, but not advised in pregnancy or breast-feeding.

Nettle
Source of iron.
Leaves, cooked or as tea.

Uses: Iron deficiency, to supply calcium. Roman soldiers used to bring nettles with them to make their skin feel warm.

Side-effects: Stings.

Parsley
Antispasmodic, alterative, source of iron.
Leaves may be chewed and eaten and the root used in an infusion.

Uses: Iron-deficiency anaemia, soothing the gut, freshening the breath. The ancient Egyptians, Greeks and Roman used it for abdominal pain and bladder problems.

Side-effects: May upset the kidneys, not to be used with kidney disease or in pregnancy. The seeds must never be taken.

Peppermint
Antispasmodic, anti-nauseant, carminative.
Leaves.

Uses: Diverticulitis, flatulence, irritable bowel symptoms. Known since the 17th century.

Side-effects: None are described but it is best avoided in pregnancy or breast-feeding.

Raspberry
Relaxant, digestive, antispasmodic.
Leaves and fruit.

Uses: In chronic diarrhoea, colic, to relax the womb.

Side-effects: None listed.

Rosemary
Digestive, nerve tonic, hepatic.
> May be taken as tea, an infusion to relieve depression and headache associated with stomach upset.
> Side-effects: May make migraine worse if taken during an attack.

Sage
Tonic, nerve tonic, febrifuge.
> Leaves.
> Uses: To stimulate appetite, to help with flatulence and grief and protect against infection (viral). In 1597 Gerard wrote that 'it quickeneth the senses and memory, strengtheneth the sinews, and restoreth health to those with shakey trembling of the members.' It has a reputation for giving long life - even immortality.
> Side-effects: None described.

Senna
Stimulant laxative.
> Pods and leaves are used.
> Uses: For moderately severe constipation, frequently added to herbal remedies to increase their efficacy.
> Side-effects: Griping, but less than most stimulant laxatives.

Skullcap
Restorative, nerve tonic.
> Leaves made into tea.
> Uses: For convalescents, to cope with stress. At one time used for rabies.
> Side-effects: None described.

St John's Wort
Nervine, antidepressant, nerve tonic.
> Flowers, leaves.
> Uses: Mild and moderate depression. It has an action like fluoxetine - Prozac. Used to be considered a protection against ghosts, spirits and witchcraft.
> Side-effects: Interacts with other antidepressants and medicines for high blood pressure: rash. Not for severe depression.

Siberian Ginseng
Nerve tonic, nervine, sedative.

Uses:	In convalescence, poor sleep, stress and anxiety. Was used by the Russians for their astronauts.
Side-effects:	Breast discomfort, heavy periods (milder than Korean and Chinese ginseng).

Slippery Elm
Demulcent, nutritive.
Inner part of the bark is used.

Uses:	To soothe an upset digestive system, especially with diverticulitis, and makes a suitable first food after a liquid diet.
Side-effects:	None.

Valerian
Nervine, sedative, laxative - 'God's Valium'.
Leaves.

Uses:	Calming in anxiety and depression, helps with sleep, helps with irritable bowel symptoms, especially when constipation is a problem.
Side-effect:	In some people can make their anxiety worse.

Willow
Febrifuge, restorative, anti-nauseant, anti-inflammatory.
Bark used before cinchona (quinine came from this) in malaria and other fevers.
Uses: Chronic diarrhoea, nausea, poor digestion, recurrent fever, pain.
Side-effects: Upset stomach.

Recommended Herbs for Specific Symptoms of Diverticular Disease

Flatulence and bloating –	Peppermint, sage, fennel.
Diarrhoea –	Yellow dock, cinnamon, ginger, raspberry leaf tea.
Constipation –	Dandelion root, aloe vera root.
Stress and pain –	Valerian, camomile, slippery elm.

Chapter Thirteen

Exercise

Few of us take enough exercise. Since we are only 2 per cent brain and most of the rest is bone and muscle, it figures that physical activity is natural and necessary to our bodily well-being - and that includes the health of our bowels, for those at risk of diverticulitis.

General Exercise

Exercise is good for the muscles themselves and practice improves their strength and efficiency. The abdominal muscles are particularly relevant to diverticular disease. The miserable symptoms of constipation and uncomfortable bloating are definitely improved by exercise.

Other parts that benefit are the bones, in the fight against osteoporosis, and the joints, to help with arthritis and prevent avoidable loss of mobility. Because you breathe more deeply when you take exercise, the lungs benefit and incidentally the upper air passages and sinuses, and the oxygen supply is revved up throughout. Exercise makes your heart beat faster, improving the circulation - to the brain, the toes and fingers and all the hidden, internal organs, such as the intestines. The colon, oddly, can suffer from *ischaemia* - a shortage of blood due to the arteries silting up.

Walking - There is a huge range of suitable activities to choose from but the cheapest, most useful and easiest to achieve, requiring no special apparatus or venue, is walking. A brisk daily walk for half-an-hour is probably the best tonic you can give to your body - and offers a chance to clear your mind, too.
Jogging and running - These are good, if you are young and fit enough, but they tend to jar the lower limb joints.
Swimming - Swimming is especially good for the abdominal muscles - you can feel them stretching out in the water, but you need a well-heated local pool.
Ball games - From tennis to football, ball games combine fresh air with exercise, while indoors there is table tennis, badminton or squash. The snag is that they are likely to be too strenuous when you reach the diverticular years.
Cycling - May be unsuitable for the same reason as ball games. It is an effective form of exercise for the leg and thigh muscles.

Aerobics, step-exercise and yoga - These forms of exercise may appeal to you, and so long as you are comfortable, will do you nothing but good.

Free-standing Exercises

These keep you supple. They are a healthy way to greet the day, and another 10-15 minutes before bed improves your sleep. You can combine them with watching TV or listening to the radio - or music. Aim at repeating each exercise ten times, but start with however many you can manage without strain.

● Stand on tiptoe, without shoes.
● Nod and turn your head from side to side - but avoid rolling it, which from middle age can cause you to nip a nerve.
● Alternately bend and straighten your knees in a standing position.
● With legs straight and slightly apart, bend to each side, then twist your body round to face that side.
● Touch your toes or as near as you can.
● Windmill your arms, one at a time.
● Lift your arms from your sides until they are vertical, then clasp your hands behind your head and pull your elbows backwards.
● Shrug your shoulders.
● Sit in a chair and lift up each knee until your thigh is against your abdomen.
● Sit down in a low chair and stand up - no hands.
● Standing up, swing each leg out to the side, then backwards and forwards.

Exercises You Can Do on Your Bed
These are especially useful when you are recovering from an operation.

Lying on your back:
● Pull your buttocks together.
● Straighten your abdomen, hips and knees and hold them rigid briefly.
● Bicycle your legs.
● Lift each straight leg in turn.
● Lift each leg, bending hip and knee so that your thigh is against your abdomen.
● Lift your head and shoulders off the bed and hold for a few moments.
● Sit-ups - sit up from lying flat.
● Leg-ups - lift both legs together a foot or two and slowly lower.
Lying on your front:
● Lift each straight leg off the bed in turn.

- Bend your knees with your feet in the air, then rotate your ankles clockwise and anti-clockwise.

Exercises Specifically for the Abdominal Muscles

To strengthen the abdominal muscles and help control distension, do these exercises twice a day, but not less than an hour after a meal, to achieve progressive muscle development. You are in training.

Start by doing each exercise once or twice, but build up to 10-20 repeats.

- Lie on your back, hands on your lower abdomen. Raise your legs slowly about 18 inches, with knees straight. Hold for a count of 5.
- Lie on your back, arms spread, hands pressing the floor. Raise your legs to the vertical then separate them as widely as you can, then close, pressing knees and ankles together. Repeat three times, then lower your legs and relax.
- Lie on your back, with your feet anchored under a piece of furniture if necessary, hands pressing your lower abdomen. Sit up slowly, then slowly relax.
- From the same starting position, raise your head and shoulders off the floor, turn to left and right, then return to the starting position and relax.
- Sit in a chair with a high back, with your head and shoulders against it. Gently press your lower abdomen and move your head and shoulders forwards and back again. Repeat 5 times and relax.
- Deep breathing, using your diaphragm. Pull in your abdomen strongly as you breathe in, release it as you breathe out.

Bowel Exercise

Taking up the squatting position triggers reflex peristaltic movements in the large bowel - these are waves of muscular contraction massaging the motions in the colon towards the rectum. This in turn sets off another reflex - deliberate relaxation of the anal sphincter, the double ring of muscle at the exit of the digestive system, normally keeping it shut. Modern toilets are planned for us to sit high, legs together - a position that discourages bowel activity.

To set off the reflexes and help your bowel to act, use these ploys:

- Use telephone directories, bricks or books to raise your feet 3-4 inches (7-8 cm) off the floor when you are sitting on the toilet.
- Place your feet apart.
- Bend forward to bring your abdomen against your thighs.

- With your hands above your anus, separate your buttocks while contracting your abdominal muscles, hold for a few seconds. Repeat rhythmically for 10 minutes or until a movement occurs.

Do the bowel exercise morning and evening.

If a motion is ready but seems stuck, use a plastic glove or finger stall, moisten with soap or KY jelly, insert into the anus and circle it slowly and gently just inside.

Chapter Fourteen

Psychological Aspects

There are those who will state that diverticular disease is psychosomatic. Of course it is not. There is no way that you can say an abscess or a perforation is 'all in the mind'.

However, every illness is psychosomatic in that it has a psychological and a physical side which are indivisible. And that certainly applies to diverticular disease.

The digestive system and the emotions are particularly intimately linked. Babies are born hungry and thirsty - even water is welcome for starters, and very soon they express their discontent, ranging to fury, if their stomachs are registering Empty. Contentment means a tummy filled with warm milk. During the next few years your child will say he has a 'tummy ache' if he is feeling sad - it takes longer for children to distinguish between abdominal sensations and emotional distress.

In a study of 96 children attending a clinic complaining of abdominal pain only in 13 was there a recognizable physical cause. The score was not much higher for a group of adults.

What Is the Explanation?

If you have suffered some excessive stress - such as a bereavement, moving to another country, starting a new job or long-term strain looking after an invalid partner - you may react with a depressive illness or an anxiety state. If you have a weak spot physically that, too, will be lit up in reaction to the adverse situation. Pain, in particular, is likely to get much worse. Since it is always more acceptable to mention physical symptoms, including pain, your subconscious shifts the emotional suffering onto the practical side. Bodily symptoms increase but your mood improves - you come over as brave and deserving of sympathy. If you say that you feel low, or worried, the chances are that, after a short time, other people will see you as a moaner and you yourself will feel ashamed that you cannot snap out of it.

Depression

Sufferers of depression often down-play their psychological symptoms. The give away symptoms of an underlying depression are as follows:
- Unrefreshing sleep, often waking much too early.

- Loss of energy, physical and mental.
- Loss of interest in work and all the activities you normally enjoy.
- Dulling of your emotions including love for your nearest and dearest.
- Nothing gives you the slightest cheer.
- Loss of taste - food tastes like sawdust. This may result in your not eating and losing weight - or you may chomp away automatically, even putting on weight.
- Sex leaves you cold.
- Your concentration is zilch. You find yourself reading the same paragraph over and over - you are slowed down in everything you do.
- Your eyes, skin and hair look dull and lustreless.
- Low, hopeless mood. You may feel guilty for no reason.

These symptoms, because they are so negative and unattractive, do not catch other people's sympathy. In fact, when you are bereft of your normal vitality you may come over as dreary and selfish. The mention of physical symptoms by contrast arouses instant concern - pain especially. Other people think they cannot be psychological and that there must be a physiological or practical reason for them.

Any major loss or humiliation has an impact on your immunity system. Your defences go down, leaving you vulnerable to attack from microbes or the rogue cells of cancer. If your gut is your Achilles heel and you already have a few diverticula - likely from age 45 - an infection may start up in one of them. This causes an attack of diverticulitis. It may be mild and evanescent, the beginning of a series, or severe. Complications are more likely to crop up if you are under stress and your body and mind are having to grapple with it.

Hannah's husband Simon died suddenly from a stroke. He was only 65, two years older than Hannah. She had relied on Simon for dealing with all their financial affairs, and truth to tell, he had always made the important decisions. Everyone was impressed with how well Hannah was coping after his death. However, she had pain in her lower abdomen which seemed to be connected with increasingly obstinate constipation.

Hannah had probably had 'silent' diverticulosis for years, without symptoms, but her colon was not suffering in silence now. The bereavement would have upset her immune system and now she developed full-blown diverticulitis with raised temperature, acute abdominal pain and distension. The doctor prescribed antibiotic capsules (co-trimoxazole - Septrin) and advised her to stay in bed for two or three days on a semi-liquid diet. She had also to drink more than usual, and her choice of lemon barley water was a good one: fizzy drinks, pure fruit juice, coffee and tea can irritate the sick gut.

Hannah's symptoms died down over the next seven to ten days - apart from the pain, which was always present and, if anything, worse. There was no other sign of infection now, so the doctor questioned her in detail about other symptoms and feelings. There were several pointers to a depressive illness.

- Waking early and being unable to get back to sleep.
- Concentration so poor that she could not remember what had been said a few moments before.
- Loss of appetite, loss of interest - nothing seemed worthwhile.
- Inability to feel the slightest pleasure.

Like most people in these circumstances, Hannah was offended when the doctor told her that it was an understandable depression underlying the continuing pain and that she needed an antidepressant. Nevertheless, after two weeks on a well-tried antidepressant of the tricyclic family, dothiepin (Prothiaden) she found that she was sleeping much better, and the pain was dulling down for the first time. St. John's Wort, a herbal remedy, is a moderately strong antidepressant, with a stimulating action similar to that of fluoxetine (Prozac). If Hannah had been especially keen to have a 'natural' treatment, this would have been suitable.

Since she could now manage a more substantial diet it was time to deal with her constipation. Constipation is anyway a symptom of depression, since everything is slowed down, including the activity of the gut. As the depression lifted this improved, too - with a little help from a fortnight's course of lactulose. A herbal laxative such as aloe vera might have been used, but it is more difficult to work out the dosage.

If her symptoms had been more serious she would have needed antibiotics by injection and possibly nourishment through a vein for the first few days. Any complication - bleeding, abscess, perforation - would have landed her in hospital, and the antidepressant would not have been relevant until the severe physical symptoms had abated. As it was, Hannah recovered completely from her attack of diverticulitis, including the lingering abdominal pain, and the depression never got out of control. She continued on the antidepressant, for a full nine months as recommended, at the end of which she had come through the acute phase of missing Simon.

Anxiety State

Depression is the most common response to stress, but an anxiety state runs a close second. Often the illness includes features of both.

Symptoms of an Anxiety State

- Difficulty in getting off to sleep, waking on and off all night - and feeling ready to sleep at getting-up time.
- Restlessness in the day, too - cannot settle to anything.
- Lack of concentration.
- Tense muscles - they may ache, including a colicky colon.
- Loss of appetite.
- Trembling hands and sometimes head.
- Fast heart rate, palpitations.
- Passing water frequently.
- Loose motions.
- Sweating.
- Anxious, irritable mood.
- You feel exhausted but cannot relax.

Physical sensations are sharper when you are anxious, but they are less likely to suppress the emotional symptoms than when you are in a depression.

Arnie's 50th year was the most stressful ever. He had been gazumped over a house purchase so that he and his family had to perch in rented accommodation until they found another property they could afford. His wife was not happy and inclined to blame him. Money was uncomfortably tight. Arnie developed an anxiety state which showed in a short fuse, an inability to finish any job he started and incessant worrying.

Arnie had already experienced a couple of episodes of diverticulitis, and whenever he was emotionally upset he would develop diarrhoea as he did now. It was not long before his temperature went up and he had increasingly painful colic. A check of his white cells showed he had a leucocytosis, a tell-tale sign of infection, so he was into diverticulitis and at risk of the complications.

The medicines which helped Arnie were the antibiotic ciprofloxacine (Ciproxin), which is especially helpful in pelvic infections, and the sleeping drug zopiclone (Zimovane). This he could take for a maximum of four weeks, although it is less likely to cause dependence than the older benzodiazepine compounds. He was also prescribed an antispasmodic, dicyclomine (Merbentyl), and an anxiolytic (anti-anxiety drug), buspirone (Buspar), which helped a little. Like zopiclone, buspirone is a modern medicine, not as addictive as earlier anxiolytics such as Valium.

To start with, Arnie had an anti-diarrhoeal, loperamide (Imodium), but only long enough to bring the motions under control since his doctor did not want to switch him into constipation. Arnie still likes to have a few tablets of loperamide or diphenoxylate (Lomotil) by him, so that he can check any looseness straight away. Herbal remedies for anxiety include valerian or camomile, and for diarrhoea, ginger or raspberry-leaf tea.

In Arnie's case it was the counselling that helped him most over the long term.

Counselling and Psychotherapy
Both depression and anxiety states respond to the talking treatments - counselling and psychotherapy.

Counselling
The essence of counselling is the chance to tell a sympathetic listener all that you are feeling and suffering, your hopes and fears and your background - and hearing some common-sense answers. The counsellor can be a doctor, but is often a nurse or social worker who has had the appropriate training.

For complex and severe cases when the emotional aspects are disabling, it is essential to have the assistance of a psychiatrist or clinical psychologist.

Psychotherapy
This can be carried out in groups, when it is most effective for chronic conditions, but it is usually offered on a one-to-one basis. There is a whole range of therapies to choose from, with cognitive and analytical therapies at opposite poles.

Cognitive Therapy
This is based on reasoning of the Socratean style, in which the client is guided to work out for himself which patterns of thought are liable to encourage his symptoms, and to help him to rid himself of those which have become a bad habit. Six to ten sessions are usually enough.

Analytical Psychotherapy
Analytical psychotherapy, by contrast, may continue for two years and involves a deep and far-reaching examination of the personality and why it has developed as it has. The object is to understand the symptoms, as well as other aspects of the subject's life.

The purpose of counselling and psychotherapy in diverticular disease is to consider the whole person, mind as well as body.

Personality
Diverticular disease can present in different ways, for some resembling the irritable colon syndrome, with its multiple, variable symptoms, for others

with a constant tendency to constipation, or with diarrhoea as a key problem. Often, which symptoms predominate is a matter of personality.

Introverts
Introverts usually want control. When this is applied to diverticular disease it means tightening of the gut muscles, like clenching a fist. It leads to constipation, steady pain and in severe cases can contribute to obstruction. Obsessional people, who have difficulty in letting go of their feelings, are equally inhibited about releasing their motions when they are stressed or anxious.

Whatever your personality, there will be times when you feel yourself tensing up, feeling stressed, worn out or unduly down. It is worthwhile taking a few minutes to try and shift gear.

Quick-Fix
1. Stretch like a cat - arms, legs and back as far as they will go in each direction.
2. Oxygenate your brain and your body with half a dozen slow, deep breaths, using your ribs and your diaphragm.
3. Close your eyes and with each breath out, say whatever you want to be true. For example:
   ● I've got by so far - I can cope with anything fate throws at me.
   ● Most people like me and wish me well.
   ● If anyone else can do it - I can.
   ● I am a really worthwhile person.
4. Zap any sneaky thoughts about difficulties, failure, worry. Substitute an up-beat one.
5. Ball your fists than splay your fingers out a few times.
6. Give someone else a lift - with a phone call, a postcard or an e-mail containing a parcel of praise.

Chapter Fifteen

Eating for Health

Eating can and should be a pleasure to look forward to and enjoy three or four times a day - an intake of the stuff of life, and a top social activity. Fast foods, pasta, chips and chocolate are tasty, convenient - and cheap. They are also no good for your colon. On the other hand, too much meat, saturated fat, sugar and alcohol are also harmful - and that is not the worst: *SMOKE ALARM*: Cigarettes damage your digestive tract, and specifically your colon.

You may suffer from constipation or its opposite, distension or discomfort in the abdomen, and the middle-aged spread. That is your colon crying out for the natural foods for which it was designed. It may mean retraining your appetite to appreciate a high-fibre diet based on fresh fruit and salads, vegetables cooked and raw, whole-grain cereals, wholemeal and nuts - plus enough meat, fish, egg or cheese to fulfil your need for protein, which will probably be less than you think.

You cannot bolt raw foods and others rich in fibre as you could a chunk of cake or a burger in a bun - your digestion will not play. So you must allot a minimum of 15 minutes, peaceful eating time for each meal - whether at your desk, in a café or canteen, or on a corner of the kitchen table at home. If you are alone, and inclined to rush, reading while you eat slows the pace and takes your mind away from current worries.

Regular High-fibre Diet

A high-fibre diet is what you need if you have diverticular disease, or want to prevent its developing. It is good for your general health, and an anti-cancer choice, too.

Daily Plan
On Waking
Glass of hot water, weak tea or coffee (coffee may be too strong on an empty stomach).
Breakfasts
Drinks with every breakfast:
- Fruit juice - optional, small quantity.
- Herb tea, tea, coffee or low-fat chocolate, preferably after rather than during the eating.

- Porridge (oats or bran cereal) with stewed fruit, prunes or sliced banana and milk.
- Muesli and milk, fresh or stewed fruit.
- Three fresh fruits, e.g. plum, pear, orange, apple, banana, kiwi, peach; 2-3 rye crispbreads.
- Whole grapefruit, wholemeal toast with spread and honey (on the comb if possible).
- Stewed fruit or sliced fresh fruit and yoghurt. Brown or wholemeal toast or crispbread.
- Grilled bacon, tomatoes and mushrooms with crusty wholemeal bread. Boiled or poached egg or cold ham may substitute for the bacon.

Elevenses
- Tea, coffee, apple juice.
- Piece of fruit, raw carrot or celery.

Lunches
Water or still mineral water before and a little with the meal if needed.
  Coffee or tea or herb tea, e.g. peppermint, to follow the meal.
  Choose from:
- Vegetable soup with plenty of chopped fresh vegetables and barley (onion, celery, carrot, parsnip, broccoli, aubergine, green beans, peppers - plus peas, beans and lentils only if you do not have any problems with wind or bloating). Wholemeal roll or oatcake and cheese. Apple.
- Sardines or scrambled egg with parsley on wholemeal toast. Tomato salad. Banana.
- Potato in its jacket, with tuna, cheese or ham filling. Salad. Fresh fruit and fromage frais.
- Tuna, egg, chicken, cheese, ham or sardine salad. Crisp brown roll. (Lettuce, peppers, cucumber, tomatoes, beetroot, grated carrot and any cold vegetables.)

Teas
Tea, herb tea, coffee, juice.
  Optional: Piece of fruit.
  Cucumber or tomato sandwich.
  Marmite and lettuce on crispbread.

Suppers
Choose from:
- Meat, fish or poultry - any. Large helping of salad or vegetables including potatoes. Oatcake and cheese.

- Cauliflower cheese with two vegetables. Fresh fruit.
- Herb or mushroom omelette and grilled tomatoes. Fruit flan.
- Mixed vegetable casserole sprinkled with cheese, cress or watercress, and granary roll. Baked apple with sultanas and ice-cream.
- Stir-fried chicken and vegetables. Fruit sorbet.
- Vegetable curry and brown rice. Stewed or fresh fruit and yoghurt.

Water or still mineral water with the meal.
Coffee, herb tea or tea to follow.

Late Evening
Glass of hot water.
Slippery elm drink.
Choose cakes, biscuits and puddings which contain dried fruit, carrot, nuts and coconut.

Alcohol
Not more than two alcoholic drinks a day - a drink means a small sherry, half-a-pint of lager or beer, a small glass of wine, or a pub measure of spirits. Drink extra water if you take alcohol.

Quantities
A standard helping of breakfast cereal is three heaped tablespoons, and of porridge four level tablespoons.

A portion of meat, fish, etc. is 3-4 oz (100-120 g)
Portion of cheese as an extra 2-3 oz (80 g)

Normal daily intake:
At 45:   for a man 2,000 kcals,   1,800 for a woman
At 60:   for a man 1,900 kcals,   1,700 for a woman
At 80:   for a man 1,800 kcals,   1,600 for a woman

Checks and Balances
Fibre - Ensure that you are having at least three fibre-rich foods daily - see the list on p. 116.
Vitamins and minerals - These are vital to your health, and the diet suggested provides these special factors. An excess can be harmful, but this is unlikely if you take all you need through your food. The only vitamins in which you may run low are vitamin C, folate, and of the minerals - iron and calcium.

Water-soluble Vitamins

Vitamin C (Ascorbic Acid)
Good in infection, for the immune system and brainwork, and the skin.

Where to find it - Fresh fruit, especially blackcurrants and citrus fruits, salads and rapidly boiled vegetables (canning and freezing do not cause much loss).

Thiamin (B1)
Enables us to make use of carbohydrate foods, our main source of energy. Heavy drinkers cannot absorb it properly.

Where to find it - Whole wheat, pulses, nuts, pork, Marmite. White bread and rice use up excessive amounts of this vitamin, and raw fish destroys it.

Niacin
Needed by the digestive and breathing systems.

Where to find it - Liver, kidneys, Marmite, beef extract, eggs - and instant coffee. Tablets of nicotinic acid make the skin flush and are sometimes given to pep up the circulation in chilblains.

Riboflavin
Enables the body to make the best use of its oxygen supply. As with thiamin, the amount you need depends on how much food there is requiring processing.

Where to find it - The usual sources are liver, cheese and eggs, but meat and yeast extracts have higher concentrations.

Vitamin B12 (Cobalamin)
Vital for making red blood corpuscles and a deficiency causes pernicious anaemia, with dire effects on the nervous system.

Where to find it - B12 is unique in that it is not found in any plant. Vegetarians get their supplies from milk, eggs and cheese. Other sources are meat and poultry and especially liver. Strict vegans are likely to run into trouble. A parasite in raw fish (for example in Sushi) can use up our supply, and some medicines, for instance colchicine and slow-release potassium, prevent its absorption.

Folic Acid
A lack causes a form of anaemia, with weakness and tiredness. It crops up in older people living on their own with a tea-and-biscuits diet, and those who live on rice. Hormone replacement therapy, anti-epileptic drugs and too much alcohol interfere with its absorption.

Where to find it - Liver, broccoli, savoy cabbage, beans and oranges. Cooking tends to destroy it.

Vitamin B6 (Pyridoxine)
All-round usefulness to the metabolism. No one runs short of this except, rarely, if they are taking an anti-tuberculosis drug, or oestrogen, as in hormone replacement therapy. The danger lies in taking too much, as tablets. This can make you ill.

Where to find it - Cereals, meat, green vegetables and fruits.

Fat-soluble Vitamins

Vitamin A (Retinol)
For night vision and your skin.

Where to find it - Milk, butter, spread, cheese, egg yolk, liver. Its precursor, beta-carotene, from which your body can make it, is found in carrots, green vegetables, sweet potatoes and apricots. It is destroyed by sunlight, for instance in dried apricots, but protected by Vitamin E. Excess intake, from fish-liver oils, is more likely to cause symptoms than a lack of it.

Vitamin D
The sunshine vitamin. It enables the body to absorb calcium for the bones, and is normally manufactured from the oils of the skin by the action of sunlight. A dark skin is a disadvantage for this.

Where to find it - Fish-liver oils and herrings, including kippers, and in small quantities in sardines, spread and eggs. Some elderly people who have to spend all their time indoors may need Vitamin D tablets, with milk and cheese to provide calcium. An excess is dangerous, and harmful to the arteries.

Vitamin K
Necessary for the blood to clot.

Where to find it - Fresh, green leafy vegetables - but there is little likelihood of running short unless you are seriously ill, or on antibiotics for a long time with a poor diet.

Vitamin E
An anti-cancer vitamin with several ill-defined uses.

Where to find it - Wheatgerm, sunflower seeds, palm and other polyunsaturated oils, spreads. You will not run short on an ordinary diet.

Minerals

Only two minerals are important in the age group when diverticular disease is rife.

Calcium
Necessary for the health of your bones and to ward off osteoporosis, also for nerve and muscle function. Those most at risk of running low are women after the menopause and anyone taking steroids or on an inadequate diet.

Where to find it - Hard cheeses, milk, sardines, white flour in the UK, where it is fortified with calcium. A trap in modern eating is to take exclusively wholemeal or brown flour products.

Iron
A key constituent of haemoglobin, the red pigment in blood, transporting oxygen to all parts of the body. Lack of iron from even minor blood loss, or an inadequate diet, leads to iron-deficiency anaemia, the most common type. Up to 20 per cent of over-sixties are anaemic.

Where to find it - Liver, meat (not fish), eggs, All-bran, treacle, dried fruit and dark chocolate. Green vegetables, despite their reputation, are not a worthwhile source of iron, but Vitamin C in fresh fruit and raw vegetables aids its absorption. So does alcohol. Iron tablets are a cheap, effective treatment for anaemia, but may cause constipation or diarrhoea.

Zinc is worth mentioning only because, although it is fashionable, it is of no practical importance except for chronic alcoholics, or those who take enormous quantities of bran.

Where to find it - Oysters, wholemeal, meat.

Convalescence

This is the end-stage of successful recovery, but you are still mentally and physically depleted. Your body and mind will need time to pick up.
- Have frequent breaks in whatever you are doing - never force yourself to carry on, but wait until you feel ready.
- Don't miss out on meals, particularly breakfast and lunch. They need not be big meals but should each include some easily digested carbohydrate, from slippery elm to rich tea biscuits to porridge.
- Watch your bowels - drink plenty of water.
- Have a change of scene once or twice a day.
- Have a daily 'fix' of exercise, and of fresh air.
- See friends, especially those who can make you laugh.

- Wind down in the evening with TV, reading or music.
- Don't stay up late, but don't go to bed at nursery time - 10.30 is reasonable.

Convalescent Diet
Avoid temporarily:
- Alcohol, tea, coffee, cola, meat-extract drinks and fizzy minerals.
- Pickles, curries, spices.
- Fried or twice-cooked foods.
- Sausages, bacon, pork.
- Fatty fish such as sardines, mackerel, herrings.
- New bread, wholemeal.
- Excess of sugar and sweets, chocolate.
- Raw vegetables.
- Dried fruit, nuts, tomatoes and unpeeled fruit.

Hurry through anything else, but eat in an oasis of tranquillity. It need not take long. Whatever and whenever we eat, each meal or snack is a relief from mental or physical strain, and when it is shared it is an affirmation of friendship or love.

Appendix

A Brief Medical History of Diverticular Disease

The Egyptians: we know from their papyri that disorders of the bowel were well recognized as early as 2000 BC. The Ebers papyrus (1700 BC) lists 33 prescriptions for 'injections' into the back passage, including honey, myrrh and ibex fat. Enemas, suppositories and purges were commonplace treatments.

The Greeks: the writings of Hippocrates (460-370 BC) include sections on piles and fistulae, with directions for surgery, while Herodotus remarks on the necessity for specialists in colo-rectal disease.

The Romans: copied the Greeks, but added little themselves. In the 1st century AD the emperor Claudius passed laws regulating when it was appropriate to fart. After the Romans there followed the Dark Ages, when more knowledge was lost than advanced.

St Fiacre, a Christian of the 7th century, became the patron saint of diseases of the bowels and of gardeners. A hostelry in Paris was named after him, and the carriages standing outside came to be called 'fiacres'.

Medical progress was slow in the Middle Ages.

John of Arderne, in the 14th century, was a surgeon specializing in diseases of the bowel, and he wrote a treatise on 'ileal passion', meaning obstruction of the bowel. He is also remarkable for charging such enormous fees that patients often had to pay by an annuity; this enabled him to treat poor people free.

William Harvey, who worked out, in the 17th century, how the blood circulated, pointed out the sympathetic connection between the bowels and the psyche. 'The belly is the counterpart of the face,' he wrote: each reflects the emotions. Most medical research work took place at Salerno, in Italy, at this time, and Sir John Harington, a godson of Queen Elizabeth, translated a relevant passage:

'Great Harmes have grown and Maladies exceeding,
By keeping in a little blast of wind:
So cramps and dropsy, colics have their breeding,
And mazed brains, for want of vent behind.'

Perhaps he was thinking of bloating.

Learning was again advancing.

Dr Alexis Littré of Paris published, in 1710, the first anatomically accurate description of diverticular disease. He had examined a dead baby with a malformed gut, which ended in a cul-de-sac. He followed this up with autopsies on adults and in some, he found what he considered to be hernias of the bowel - the blind-ended saccules we call diverticula. Littré also envisaged, but did not carry out, the procedure of *colostomy*, a frequently performed operation today. It comprises making an artificial exit from the colon in the abdomen, usually because of an obstruction.

Littré was followed by Matthew Baillie, who wrote a great work in 1793: *The Morbid Anatomy of Some of the Most Important Parts of the Human Body.* He included the bowel and mentioned diverticular disease under the name of *scirrhus of the sigmoid colon*. This is the area where nearly all diverticular disease develops. Post-mortem examinations were now made on anyone of note whose illness was interesting. Dr Johnson was one such.

The 19th century: this period was as remarkable as our own for the flood of new knowledge - unravelling old problems and breaking new ground in science, technology and medicine. All the great doctors of the day contributed something to the information about diverticular disease, among them Cruveilhier, Klebs and Koch on the continent, and William Cripps in England. In 1888 Cripps introduced the operation of *colotomy*: cutting into the colon to drain an abscess, which might well have developed in a diverticulum.

1895: Wilhelm Roentgen discovered X-rays, sparking a revolution in diagnosis for those areas, like the chest and abdomen, which are normally hidden. It was not immediately relevant to diverticular disease, since soft tissues do not show up without assistance.

1902: diseases of the bowel were made not only respectable but fashionable when Sir Frederick Treves operated on Edward VII for acute appendicitis. The appendix, after all, is only a normal diverticulum and acute diverticulitis has often been called 'left-sided appendicitis'. The symptoms are similar, but on the left side instead of the right. It was at about this time that the term *gastroenterology* came into use, conferring dignity on the practitioners of stomach and bowel disease.

1904: Dr A. Schule produced an enema that was opaque to X-rays and showed up the outline of the colon.

1908: Sir Arthur Hurst developed the technique to demonstrate in detail the mechanics of the colon, the passing of motions, and constipation. Later he founded a gut doctors' club which became the British Society of Gastroenterology.

1914: De Quervain and Costa showed X-ray pictures of actual diverticula of the colon by the use of an improved barium enema. This opened a new era.

The Age of Technology
This has shaped modern gastroenterology and specifically caused the colon to give up its secrets. It was well under way 200 years ago.

1806: Borrini invented the first *endoscope* - a tube pushed into the back passage, to give a sight of the inside.

1904: Lockhart-Mummery in England introduced the electric endoscope, in the case of the bowel a *sigmoidoscope*, but it was limited in reach and extremely uncomfortable.

1952-1954: Professor Harold Hopkins set to work to make a fully flexible sigmoidoscope in which the light travelled along glass fibres which were also flexible: fibreoptics. Since then, most of the work on endoscopes has been led by the Japanese.

1957: Professor Matsunaga of Hirohito University developed cameras for use in endoscopy.

1969: his colono-fibroscope, now called a colonoscope, became available commercially.

Useful Addresses

United Kingdom

British Colostomy Association
15 Station Road
Reading
Berkshire RG1 1LG

British Society of Gastroenterology
3 St Andrew's Place, Regents Park
London NW1 4LB
Tel: 020 7387 3534
Fax: 020 7487 3534
email: bsg@mailbox.ulcc.ac.uk
website: http://www.bsg.org.uk

Digestive Disorders Foundation
3 St Andrew's Place, Regents Park
London NW1 4LB
Tel: 020 7486 0341
Fax: 020 7224 2012
email: ddf@digestivedisorders.org.uk.
website: http://www.digestivedisorders.
org.uk

Irritable Bowel Syndrome Network
St John's House
Hither Green Hospital
London SE13 6RU

USA

American College of Gastroenterology
4900B South 31st Street
Arlington, VA 22206
Tel: (703) 820-7400
Fax: (703) 931-520
website: http://www.acg.gi.org/ct.home.
html

*American Digestive Health
Foundation (ADHF)*
7910 Woodmont Avenue, 7th Floor
Bethesda, MD 20814 - 3015
Tel: (301) 654-2635
Fax: (301) 654-1140
email: dlee@gastro.org.
website: http://mars.gastro.org?adhf.html

National Digestive Diseases Clearinghouse
2 Information Way, Bethesda
MD 20892 - 3570
website: http://www.niddk.nih.govhealth
/digest/digest.htm

Canada

Northwestern Society of Intestinal Research
c/o Vancouver Hospital and
 Health Sciences Centre
855 W. 12th Avenue
Vancouver
BC V5Z 1M9
Tel: (604) 875-4875
Fax: (604) 875-4429
email: nsir@interchange.ubc.ca

Australia

Gastroenterological Society of Australia
145 Macquarie Street
Sydney NSW 2000
Tel: (02) 9256 5454
website: http://www.gesa.org.au

The Gut Foundation Research Institute
c/o Gastrointestinal Unit
The Prince of Wales Hospital
Randwick NSW 2031
Tel: (02) 9382 2749
Fax: (02) 9382 2828
email: gutfound@gut.nsw.edu.au

Index

127

128